THE NEW NUTRITION

MEDICINE FOR THE MILLENNIUM

Dr. Michael Colgan

YOUR PERSONAL GUIDE
TO OPTIMUM HEALTH

C.I. Publications

San Diego, 1994

For information contact: C.I. Publications, 523 Encinitas Blvd, Suite 204, Encinitas , CA 92024

FIRST EDITION

Library of Congress Cataloging-in-Publication Data
Colgan, Michael, 1939-
The New Nutrition

Bibliography:p
Includes index.
1. Health 2. Nutrition 3. Vitamins
I. Title

ISBN 0-9624840-6-7(cloth)
ISBN 0-9624840-7-5 (pbk)

Printed in the United States of America

To Lesley,
my love, my life

Also by Dr. Michael Colgan:

Electrodermal Responses

The Training Index

The Power Program

Your Personal Vitamin Profile

Prevent Cancer Now

Optimum Sports Nutrition

Sexual Potency

Forewords

"For decades, nutrition has been dishwater dull. Saturday Night live Church Chat like spokespeople soothingly reassured us that real dangers didn't exist and that no more important advances have occurred over the last half century than three squares a day. Dr. Michael Colgan leads the way in making nutrition vital and engaging. His prescriptions for change are fun and dramatically enhance personal health and fitness. My family and I use the highly motivational MEDICINE FOR THE MILLENNIUM for a better healthier life."
Dr. Bob Arnot
CBS Medical Unit.

"Michael Colgan's nutritional advice has always kept me young, fit and happy for the past fifteen years. His new book "The New Nutrition: Medicine for the Millennium" will be an invaluable resource for anyone interested in health, fitness and improving the quality of life."
Kathy Keeton
President: Omni and Longevity Magazines.

"This is a powerful book that anyone can use to learn the truth about the food we eat. This is the book about nutrition that the establishment doesn't want you to read."
Lee Labrada
International Bodybuilding Champion

"Being the chief operations officer of the largest attended professional seminars in the chiropractic profession, I have had the great opportunity to study, work with, and have available on our seminar program many of the greats in the scientific, nutritional world, includings such as Nobel Prize Winner Linus Pauling. Dr. Michael Colgan is at the top of my list. Professional nutritional researcher, author, and speaker, Dr. Colgan is held in high esteeem by our profession, and we respect his practical and informational methodologies of presenting scientifically documented nutritional information. This, his latest book, is another of his nutritonal literary masterpieces that can greatly benefit anyone who reads it."
Dr. Karl Parker
COO, Parker Chiropractic, Dallas.

"Once again Dr. Colgan has placed himself in the forefront of those pioneers in the science of nutrition. As with his previous work, he provides critical information in an easily understood, highly readable manner. This book should be read....... no, make that studied by everyone interested in optimizing their health."
Dr. David Cornsweet
Del Mar, CA.

"Thanks to Dr Mike for his wonderful expert advice. The supplements he recommended have had a big impact on my quality training. I am breaking personal records and have just won at the Nationals. I am really beginning to feel finely tuned. It's good!"
Regina Jacobs
US National 1500 meters Champion.

"Dr. Michael Colgan's books have played a major role in awakening the public - and as a consequence, the medical establishment - to the remarkable role vitamin supplements can play in enhancing health and extending life. His "New Nutrition", based on state of the art nutrition research, carries the process a giant step forward. Read it, and reap good health!"
Dr. Bernard Rimland
President, Autism Research Institute.

"Over the past decade and more, I have worked closely with Michael Colgan and have learned to respect his research tremendously. His new book entitled "The New Nutrition" is a classic book for the layman which will revolutionize the way we view nutrition and how vitamins and minerals can play an important role in combatting disease. Michael Colgan indeed presents a nutrition and lifestyle program that could well become a model for the 21st century adult (men and women). I recommend it to everyone who wants better health and increased vitality."
Ben Weider, PhD
President, International Federation of Bodybuilders.

"A definite home run! Dr. Colgan explains the latest research on nutrition, disease and our environment into a health program understandable to everyone. He is up to the minute, and entertaining."
Pete Rose
Star of the Cinncinati Reds
Holder of the record for most hits.

"In an industry cluttered with fraudulent claims, over-zealous marketers, misinformed "experts", and money hungry opportunists, it's truly a relief to know that there is a reliable resource for truth in nutrition.

It's hard to believe, after "Optimum Sports Nutrition", that there's any information left for you to cover, yet again you've done a spectacular job of making the truth readable, understandable, and valuable.

After my first reading of "The New Nutrition, Medicine for the Millennium", I realize that anyone concerned about their health and well being is left vulnerable and victimized without a copy of this revealing and insightful work.

As Americans striving for optimal performance, we need this information desperately. I beg of you, keep it coming!"
Phil Kaplan
Host of "The Mind & Muscle Fitness Hour".
Publisher of "The Health & Wealth Newsletter".

"Another exciting new book and fine contribution to nutrition science by Dr. Colgan. He is certainly one of nutritions premier authorities."
Dr. Myron Wentz
Founder of Gull Laboratories, Inc.

"With "The New Nutrition" Dr. Colgan once again meets his normal standard of excellance! This book should be entitled - Wake Up America."
Joseph Bassett
President, National Nutritional Foods Association.

"For years I have told people that lifelong fitness is a viable option. A great tool to help you on that path is provided by Dr. Colgan's book "The New Nutrition". In it, he combines the scholarship of a fine scientist with the writing skills of a novelist to weave the latest research on nutrition, disease and our environment into a health program understandable to everyone."
Bob Delmontique
Renowned fitness consultant to major corporations
Author of "Lifelong Fitness".

"Throughout my career as a Formula One and Indy Car driver, health and good nutrition have always played major roles both in my personal and professional lives. These interests - and our mutual association with Neogen - have led me to come to know Dr. Colgan. He has since helped me greatly improve my abilities, and his vast expertise of how nutrition affects the body's athletic performance easily leads all others in the field."
Eddie Cheever
Board of Directors, Neogen.
Professional Race Car Driver, Indianapolis, 1994.

"Michael has done it again!!! This book tells the truth that is needed if we are going to be able to help ourselves and our patients. We use all Michael's books for patient education and it is reassuring to know that patients are being given well tested, accurate information, instead of advertisement hype."
Dr Renè Espy, Los Angeles, CA.

"Dr. Michael Colgan has always been a major influence in modern day sports nutrition. In "The New Nutrition", he continues to inform and educate those who wish to optimize and maximize their health. If you are looking for an easy to comprehend guide to health, this book is it!"
Chris Aceto & Laura Creavalle
America's "Fittest Couple".

"A challenging and ground breaking work - how to get healthy and maintain it. Dr. Colgan quickly brings you up to speed on how to make proper nutrition work - and exposes those who would keep you from such vital health information. A great addition to "Optimum Sports Nutrition". Well documented."
Mark Scott
WXYT-AM Radio, Detroit.

"Bravo to Dr. Michael Colgan! "The New Nutrition: Medicine for The Millennium" is precise and truthful with no hype or fluff. It is highly recommended to those individuals desiring truth and knowledge.

Of all the guests interviewed on "Calling Dr. Whitaker", Dr. Michael Colgan stands head and shoulders above the majority. As a scientist, he is ethical and has a no-nonsense approach to nutrition. If you value your health, I recommend this book without reservation."
Dr. Donald R. Whitaker
Host of "Calling Dr. Whitaker", Dallas.

Acknowledgments

The wisdom of so many fine people led me to this book, I cannot hope to name them. In thanking a few I extend my thanks to all.

Stuart Slater, my mentor at Victoria University in New Zealand, taught me to become a lifetime lie-hunter, with science as my guide. Michael Brines at Rockefeller University in New York, showed me how to constantly refine my measurements because truth dwells only in the house of minute precision.

Jonas Salk, Linus Pauling, Walter Mertz and especially Renè Dubos helped me appreciate the vast design of the cosmos, and man's tiny place within it as the miraculous enlivenment of a handful of the elements of the Earth.

Roger Williams, Richard Passwater, and Carl Pfeiffer led me to realize how human beings are constantly renewing assemblages of nutrients that, if correctly provisioned, can resist all disease and live in health indefinitely.

Through all my stumbling writing, my wife and fellow scientist, Lesley, kept me firmly on track with wonderful humor and incisive analysis.

My colleagues and friends whose kind words appear in the Forewords, wrote excellent reviews and criticisms. Jeanne Soper helped tremendously with the manuscript, and Mary O'Hara with the proofing. And Kim Sawyer kept the whole book together, I know not how, through all my foibles and failings.

My thanks to everyone for making me look so good.

Introduction

This book analyses the evidence from government documents, and medical and scientific research that we have depleted our soils, contaminated our water, polluted our food and our air, degraded our food supply, mistreated our bodies, and thereby have created much of the disease that now plagues our lives.

It also reveals evidence that a large part of this degeneration has resulted from inept and iniquitous actions of certain health agencies in hidden agenda alliances with the greed of commercial enterprise, aiming to maximize power and profit at the expense of human health. America today struggles helplessly in the grip of a vast sickness industry. Government and health agencies are powerless to protect you. You have to learn to protect yourself.

The book also analyses the overwhelming evidence that, by choosing to eat the right foods and nutritional supplements, and by making simple changes in your lifestyle, you can prevent and even reverse far more disease than any doctor, any hospital, and drug, any combination of medical treatments known to man.

But remember, I am a scientist, not a physician. My 20 years of research is on nutrition, exercise, and lifestyle influences on human health, performance, and longevity. I am not trained in dispensing medical advice. That is the exclusive function of your physician. All that I am trained to do is tell you the scientific truth.

I urge you to consult the medical, scientific, and government references with which I support each inference. That way you can decide for yourself the merits of my analysis. For this is only one small book that can cover only a tiny fraction of the evidence. I have done my best to ensure that it covers a true and representative fraction. Even so, use of high dosages of nutrients and even regular exercise are still experimental health strategies. So if you choose to pursue them, you do so upon your own responsibility.

No one should exercise nor take large doses of nutrients on a continuing basis without the advice of a physician who is trained in nutrition. Some diseases can be adversely affected by nutrients and by exercise, and some nutrients can nullify the effects of certain prescribed medications.

Nevertheless, having seen profound benefits in over 32,000 people, including thousands of elite athletes who have adopted Colgan Institute programs over the last 20 years, and having seen the same health improvements in myself and my family, I urge you to examine the evidence that nutrition and exercise will become the medicine of the millennium. It could save your life.

Michael Colgan PhD.
San Diego
July 1994

Contents

Chapter 1

How Well Do You Eat?

Some uninformed medical folk still claim that a high intake of vitamins and minerals is not a magic bullet against disease. They cling to the erroneous concept of the Four Food Groups, claiming that all you need is three square meals a day from meats, dairy foods, fruits and vegetables, and grains. They also claim that, as long as you eat a variety of foods from the Four Food Groups, you need not worry about searching for whole grains, or organic vegetables, or low-fat meats and dairy foods, because our food supply is well-regulated and is the most nutritious of any country in the world. *If you want optimal health, don't believe a word of it!*

The Four Food Groups and the great nutrition provided by our food are a fraud. They were originally developed by clever commercial interests and their tame (paid) scientists for one purpose - financial gain! With no thought for human health, they have been foisted on the American public for the last 50 years.

This monumental fraud stems from the discovery of

mechanisms in the human body that motivate us to seek out and eat fat and sugar. These mechanisms likely developed in our hunter/gatherer ancestors to ensure that they ate animal fats and sweet plants whenever they got their hands on them, so they would have plentiful reserves of energy and micronutrients during the frequent times of scarcity. The same mechanisms continue in us today.

As soon as these genetically programmed appetites for fat and sugar were confirmed by science, devious industrialists looked for ways to exploit them to sell their wares. Thus the Four Food Groups were born, with meat as the first major category and dairy foods as the second. Industry quickly developed methods to breed and promote higher fat meats and to make the fattiest cheeses and creams in the world.

Fat is cheap and easy to grow into animals and, with the right promotion, can be sold v-e-e-e-ery expensive. The premium prices commanded by thickly marbled New York cuts of steak is a prime example.

Motivated by mechanisms that we call today a "sweet tooth," our ancestors sought their sugars in fruits and sweet vegetables. In that way Nature ensured that they also got all the vitamins, minerals and fiber in these natural sources. With devilish cunning and monumental ignorance of nutrition, industrial interests developed methods to extract the sugars from their nutritious sources, and to insert them into empty foods containing only excess calories.

We still have the inherited urge to eat sweet, but now most of the sweets we are offered to eat are nutritionally valueless. The sham of the Four Food Groups and the blatant lies about the nutritional value of our food supply, have turned the majority of Americans into fat and sugar processing plants to line industry's pockets.[1]

Profiteering from our inbuilt appetites would not be so bad if that was the only crime. But much worse than financial loss, the manipulation of our food has also caused untold disease and suffering. Tens of thousands of honest, but lesser educated, physicians, dieticians, social and welfare workers, teachers, and therapists have been carefully fooled into presenting supermarket foods and the Four Food Groups as correct nutrition. Many millions of Americans have followed their advice. As this book will show you, the direct result has been a massive increase in cardiovascular diseases, cancers, adult-onset diabetes, liver and kidney diseases, obesity, Alzheimers disease, arthritis, and osteoporosis.

Some physicians I have met refuse to accept the evidence that nutrition, exercise and life-style are our main defenses against disease. From the look of them I suspect they do so because they want everyone to be condemmed to the same mediocre health they suffer themselves.

Michael Colgan
Continuing Medical Education
Lectures, 1992.

Chapter 2

The Eating
Right Pyramid

Yes, I know, it sounds unbelievable that the public have been deliberately fooled into disease for 50 years, and that the real information on nutrition has been deliberately suppressed. But I am not a lone voice, a single scientist crying in the wilderness. Since I first wrote of the problem in 1982,[1] the mass of evidence that the American diet is a major cause of disease, and the huge pile of new studies that specific nutrient supplements can prevent or cure disease, have caused many thousands of health professionals to realize their error.

In April 1991, for example, the Physicians Committee for Responsible Nutrition, a Washington lobby representing 3,000 physicians, together with numerous other health organizations, demanded that the US Department of Agriculture (USDA) abandon the Four Food Groups, and reclassify meats and dairy products as "optional foods." They also demanded that the USDA recommend dramatic reductions in fat, sugar and food oil consumption.

One prominent voice, Dr. T. Colin Campbell, Professor of Nutritional Biochemistry at Cornell University, presented unequivocal evidence to the USDA, that current intakes of meat and dairy products in America are a major cause of our high rates of cancer, heart disease, diabetes, obesity, and osteoporosis. If meats and dairy products can disrupt bodily functions so much that they cause major diseases, *don't believe anyone who says they are good for you*.

Thousands of other scientists and physicians, including myself, presented similar evidence to the government, until even the most resistant politicians could no longer ignore it. But when the USDA tried to introduce the Eating Right Pyramid in 1991, the dairy, meat, sugar, and food oil lobbies screamed bloody murder. After a long fight, on 27 April 1992 America finally got a watered down version of a healthy guide to the *types* and *amounts* of different foods you should eat for optimal health.

Figure 1 shows the current USDA Eating Right Pyramid. The largest slice of the pyramid, whole grains, should form the largest part of your diet, between 30% and 45%. The next largest slice, vegetables, should be your second choice of foods, between 15% and 25% of your diet. Then comes fruits which should make up 10-15% of your diet.

Meats and dairy foods are each less than 10% of the pyramid, and should each form less than 10% of your diet. Fats, oils and sweets are the least healthy foods, and together should form only about 5% of your diet.

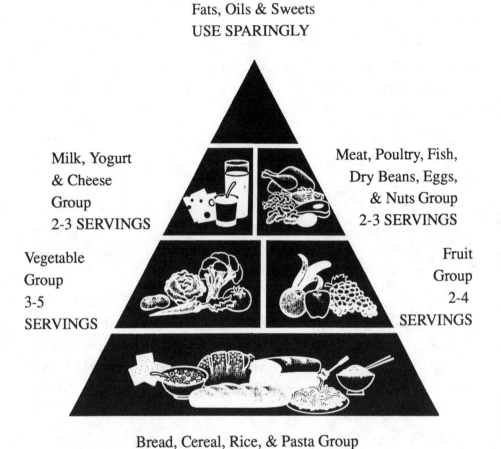

Fats, Oils & Sweets
USE SPARINGLY

Milk, Yogurt
& Cheese
Group
2-3 SERVINGS

Meat, Poultry, Fish,
Dry Beans, Eggs,
& Nuts Group
2-3 SERVINGS

Vegetable
Group
3-5
SERVINGS

Fruit
Group
2-4
SERVINGS

Bread, Cereal, Rice, & Pasta Group
6-11 SERVINGS

Figure 1. Eating Right Pyramid. Re-drawn from USDA
Publication No. 252. Hyatsville, MD : USDA, 1992.

The Pyramid Versus Our Usual Diet

Let's compare the Eating Right Pyramid with what the average American has been fooled to eat by the scam of the Four Food Groups and the supermarket food supply. Despite all the new light, lite, low-fat, no-fat foods, the USDA will tell you that the average American intake of fats and oils is still 37% of our diet.

Even if we include the high-fat meats and dairy foods, the Pyramid indicates that fat and oils should be 20-25% of your diet at most. That's what it used to be in the late 1800s before our food was degraded.[2] So one big step that the Pyramid makes towards health is to get the fat out of your food.

The next disease-bearing food is sugar. The USDA will tell you that current consumption of sugar is now 153 lbs per person per year. Average American intake of sugar has increased from 10% of our diet in the late 1800s to 65% today.[2]

The Eating Right Pyramid indicates that fruits, which are all high in sugar, should form only 10-15% of your diet. Refined sugars and sweets at the top of the Pyramid should be less than 5%. Lowering the sugar in your diet is a second big step towards health, and takes us back to about the level of sugar in the American diet of 1920.[2]

The third disease-bearing manipulation of our food is addition of extra salt and removal of natural potassium, primarily to preserve meats and dairy foods for long shelf life, and to compensate for the lack of taste in denatured, over-processed supermarket foods. Americans now eat twenty times the salt needed for optimal health.[3]

Foods in Nature, even salt-water fish, are low in sodium, high in potassium. That's what your body was designed to use. Until mass production degraded our food, the human body was never exposed to the high sodium/low potassium diet of America today. Such a diet is alien and toxic to your miraculous design.

Fresh foods are compared with processed foods in Table 1 to show how processing degrades our food. The average natural ratio for sodium to potassium in the unprocessed foods is 1 part sodium to 7 parts potassium. In the processed foods this ratio is reversed to 3.6 parts sodium to 1 part potassium.

The direct result is sodium-induced hypertension for 15 million of the 35 million hypertensives in America.[4] Hypertension is the biggest single risk for cardiovascular disease. The Pyramid helps restore potassium balance to the diet by keeping meats and dairy foods to a low proportion of your food.

The last item corrected by the Pyramid is fiber. With an emphasis on whole grains, it steers you away from white and so-called "enriched" flours and baked goods that are very low in fiber. The Pyramid steers you towards grains and breads that still retain their germ, bran and outer husk, the largest sources of beneficial fiber. As we will see, fiber, although it is not a nutrient, is essential to prevent many cardiovascular diseases and cancers.

The Eating Right Pyramid is a first step towards healthy nutrition for America. But it says nothing of the *quality* of the foods within it. Now we will see how our medical and governmental authorities, who claim responsiblity for your health, have allowed much of the food supply to become degraded and polluted to the extent that it will no longer support healthy human life.

Table 1: Sodium (Na) and Potassium (K) in Fresh and Processed Foods (mg per 100 gms).

Fresh Food	Na	K	Processed Food	Na	K
Whole wheat flour	1	120	Whole wheat bread	530	92
Round beef steak	70	400	Beef franks	1100	220
Chicken (grilled)	75	320	Chicken (canned)	495	122
Pork Loin (broiled)	66	430	Bacon	2400	390
Tuna	65	325	Tuna (canned)	800	240
Salmon	60	350	Lox	620	305
Milk (whole)	50	140	Butter	980	25
Milk (skim)	52	165	Skim cheddar cheese	725	98
Potatoes (boiled)	2	540	French fries	270	430
Asparagus	0.2	185	Asparagus (canned)	235	53
Apples	0.3	128	Apple jelly	260	190
Carrots (raw)	48	342	Carrots (canned)	245	145
Average	41	287	Average	721	200
Ratio		1:0 : 7.0	Ratio		3.6 : 1.0

Source: Colgan Institute, San Diego, CA.

Chapter 3

We Have Fouled The Land

Until the 1940s, farmers returned essential nutrients to the soil by mulching, manuring and crop rotation. These methods have worked successfully to maintain soil quality since agriculture began. But human greed and arrogance convinced commercial interests that they could use man-made technology to do better than Nature, *and make bigger profits*. So began the degradation of the American food supply.

At the end of World War II, drug conglomerates making nitrates and phosphates for weapons, were left with few buyers for their stockpiles of chemicals. They had to find new markets for their products. Earlier experiments had shown that many plants will grow on a mixture of just three minerals, nitrogen (N), phosphorus (P), and potassium (K). Armed with this knowledge, war chemical manufacturers began selling NPK fertilizers to farmers at attractive prices that made traditional soil enrichment methods uneconomic. By the '60s, in order to compete in the food market, almost all American farms had become totally dependent on NPK products in order to make a living.

Mixtures of NPK, provide three of the main minerals essential for plant health. They grow fine-looking crops with abundant yields. But your body is not a vegetable. Humans need more than nitrogen, phosphorus and potassium. They also need selenium, chromium, calcium, magnesium, iron, copper, iodine, molybdenum, zinc, cobalt, boron, and vanadium.[1] NPK fertilizers, a destructive legacy of weapons of war, do not contain the minerals essential for human health, because they were never designed for human nutrition.

As each succeeding crop grown on NPK products has depleted the soil of other essential minerals, and these minerals are no longer replaced, most produce and food animals now grown in America, have become mineral deficient. That makes you deficient also, because your body cannot make minerals and has to get them from your food.

But soil depletion is only the first assault on the American food supply. As we see in the next chapter, modern methods of food processing have also ignored Nature in favor of profit. And you are the victim.

Chapter 4

Empty Foods

Our degraded foods produced by NPK fertilizers on depleted soils are further assaulted by mass-production methods of ripening, storing, drying, cooking, freezing, blanching, pasteurization, hydrogenation, ultra-filtration and multiple other practices of modern food processing.

Don't take my word for it. The latest **RDA handbook**, itself the official government word on the quality of our food, reviews hundreds of studies, showing that the already degraded crops of today may lose even their meager supply of nutrients between harvesting and your table[1].

Here's a sample of the evidence from the **RDA handbook**:

- Vitamin E: "the tocopherol content of foods varies greatly depending on processing, storage, and preparation procedures during which large losses may occur" (p101).

- Vitamin C: "may be considerably lower because of destruction by heat and oxygen" (p117).

- Vitamin B6: "50-70% is lost in processing meats, and 50-90% is lost in milling cereals" (p144).

- (Folic acid:) "as much as 50% may be destroyed during household preparation, food processing and storage" (p150).

- (Magnesium:) "more than 80% is lost by removal of the germ and outer layers of cereal grains" (189).

Next time you eat a slice of bread, realize that the germ and outer layers of grains are removed in the making of all white and so-called "enriched" flours.

Remember, these facts are not from some scare-mongering media report. They are from the official handbook, **Recommended Dietary Allowances**, published in November 1989 by the U.S. National Academy of Sciences. They are the latest official word on nutrition.

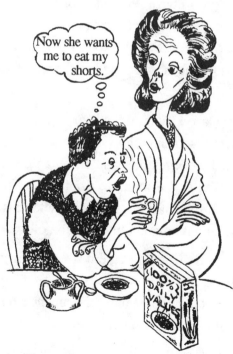

"The FDA spent $60 million of our taxes to throw out the RDA's and bring in the RDI's which are now the PDV's that everyone needs. So you are going to eat them."

More Nutrient Losses

There are volumes of other evidence showing nutrient losses by food processing. In his text, **Nutritional Evaluation of Food Processing**, Dr. Robert Harris, Professor Emeritus of Biochemistry at MIT, documents destruction of nutrients in vegetables by modern cold storage.[2] Stored grapes lose up to 30% of their B vitamins.[3] Tangerines stored for 8 weeks can lose almost half their vitamin C.[4] Asparagus stored for a week, loses up to 90% of its vitamin C.[5]

Any time you eat an apple and see the flesh turn brown within a few minutes, remember it is a sign that the apple has oxidized in storage, and has lost most of its vitamins.[6]

Dr. Theodore Labuza, Professor of Food Technology at the University of Minnesota, recently reviewed studies showing up to 90% loss of thiamin in the drying of meats[7], and losses of up to one-third of pyridoxine and pantothenic acid in freeze-drying of fish.[8]

Professor Darryl Lund of the Department of Food Science of the University of Wisconsin, shows that the process of blanching, commonly applied to vegetables and fish, can destroy one-third to one-half of their content of thiamin, riboflavin, niacin, pyridoxine, and vitamin C.[9] Similar large losses of B vitamins and vitamin C occur in the pasteurization and ultrafiltration of milk.[10]

Dr. Henry Schroeder, foremost American authority on nutrient content of foods, has shown that freezing of meats can destroy up to 50% of their content of thiamin and riboflavin, and 70% of their content of pantothenic acid.[8]

That's just a small sample of the evidence. If you add up the nutrient losses that have accrued to our food since the late 1940s, there is not a great deal left. First came degradation of the soils by use of NPK fertilizers, that do not contain the minerals essential to human health. Then came development of nutrient-poor hybrid strains of grains and vegetables that would grow better on NPK. Finally, the methods of modern food processing have stripped our food of much of its remaining nutrients. By the time it reaches your table, there is no longer any way that you can determine the nutritional value of any food you put in your mouth.

Shake and shake
the ketchup bottle,
None comes out
And then a lot'l.
Richard Armour

Chapter 5

What's Wrong With Meat?

In 1991, the Centers for Disease Control (CDC) in Atlanta released figures showing that approximately half of the 15 million pounds of antibiotics produced annually in America, are used on livestock and poultry. We have bred such sickly food animals, that in order to keep them from becoming infected, over 90% of pigs and veal calves, 60% of cattle, and 95% of all poultry have antibiotics routinely added to their feed. Residues of these drugs are in much of meat that you eat.

This over-use of antibiotics in animal feed has also bred drug-resistant strains of bacteria, which also remain in the meat you eat. The problems were first confirmed in 1986, when CDC tracked a drug-resistant strain of salmonella from an infected herd of cattle to diners who ended up in the hospital with salmonella poisoning. The deaths that resulted were given wide publicity.

Since then, following numerous outbreaks, CDC has issued public warnings that chickens and eggs may carry drug-resistant salmonella and campylobacter. These food-poisoning bacteria *kill* 2,000 Americans every year and make another six million people very ill. At least *half* of all raw chicken and eggs sold in America are contaminated.[1]

Literally hundreds of other drugs are used on livestock, and there are huge stocks of banned drugs still in use. In 1989, the pesticide **heptachlor**, banned as a carcinogen since 1978, turned up in 400,000 Arkansas chickens.

The antibacterial drug **sulfamethazine**, another known carcinogen, is a further example. Beyond a certain minimum level that will not contaminate dairy products, it is illegal for use on dairy cattle. The FDA reported in 1988 that one-quarter of all milk samples tested were contaminated with sulfamethazine.

Whenever I lecture about this drug contamination of our food, people are either outraged that government permits the crimes to continue, or they simply don't believe me. Don't take my word for it. You can confirm all these horror stories and more by calling the U.S. Department of Agriculture (USDA) Meat and Poultry Hotline, (800) 535-4555.

But don't expect the government to do anything great to protect you. Testing of meat and poultry is done by the USDA. Their own internal audit investigations show they do it very badly. Their 1988 report shows inspection errors, lost samples, incomplete testing, and allowing meats to proceed to market that should have been impounded. Overall, 78% of the meat inspection reports examined were deemed inadequate.[2] You have to protect yourself.

Healthy Meat

The free-range organically grown meat that made America great, the meat that everyone used to eat, is now a hard-to-find luxury.

With all the publicity given to organic farming and clean food, you would think the market is booming. No way. The going is tough to convert to chemical-free, low-fat livestock. The trade journal **Health Foods Business** reports that, of 59 companies who attempted to "go natural" up to 1987, less than a dozen were still in business in 1990.[3]

The big reason is cost. It is impossible to produce low-fat livestock that are free of antibiotics, hormones, and pesticides, that are also cost-competitive with mass-produced livestock. First, unlike the high-fat supermarket and hamburger livestock who spend their whole lives in small pens, organic beef need space, preferably free range. To stay lean, cattle, like people, have to exercise. They exercise by foraging. But the land they forage on has to be clean, free of pesticides. So you have a double-whammy cost of much more land per animal, and clean land too. With over 90% of America's agricultural land contaminated by pesticides, you pay an arm and a leg for any bit that isn't.

Then you need feed that is chemical free. Mary Lou Bradley, owner of B3R Country Meats, one of the best sources of clean meat, has a grain bill 10% higher than the average cattle rancher. Then, to keep the fat content of the meat at healthy levels, you have to send them to slaughter leaner. Bill Dunkleberger of Lean & Free Meats, has his beef slaughtered at 1,000 lbs, compared with 1,300 lbs for mass-produced beef. That's 300 lbs of meat per animal he doesn't get paid for. Despite these problems, there are some good sources of clean healthy meat. The best I have found are shown in Table 2.

Table 2: Natural Meats Suppliers

Beef/Veal
B3R Country Meats Inc., 2100 West Highway 287, Childress, TX 79201. (817) 937-8870.
Clean and Lean, Peach Valley Ranch, Honeywood, Ontario, Cananda. (519) 925-6628.
Coleman Natural Beef Inc., 5140 Race Court, #4, Denver, CO 80216. (303) 297-9393.
Lean & Free Products, Inc., 5265 Rockwell Drive NE, Cedar Rapids, IA 52402.

Poultry
Health is Wealth, Sykes Lane, Williamstown, NJ 08094. (609) 728-1998.
Rocky the Chicken, PO Box 1817, Sebastopol, CA 95473. (707) 829-5432.
Shelton's Poultry, 204 Loranne, Pomona, CA 91767. (909) 623-4361.
Zacky Farms, 200 N. Tyler Avenue, South El Monte, CA 91733. (800) 858-0235.

Chapter 6

Fishy Business

With all the bad reports about meat, and the salmonella contamination of poultry and eggs, fish has fast become the popular alternative source of protein. American fish consumption has increased 25% since 1980.

But it isn't all roses. In 1992, Consumers Union published results of a six-month investigation of the fish industry. They bought fish from the same places you buy it, supermarkets, grocery stores, and specialty fish shops. They sampled seven popular varieties, salmon, flounder, sole, catfish, swordfish, lake whitefish, and clams. It all smelled!

Nearly 40% of the fish were beginning to spoil at the time of purchase. Over 90% of the swordfish were contaminated with mercury. Half the whitefish and 40% of the salmon were contaminated with polychlorinated biphenyls (PCBs). The clams were laced with arsenic and lead. And this is the one that really got me: almost half of all the fish were contaminated with bacteria from *animal or human feces!*[1]

Microbiology experts reported to Consumers Union that

sewage outflows were not the source of fecal contamination of the fin fish, only the clams. The fin fish became contaminated after being caught. The report cites a litany of appalling sanitary practices during handling, processing, and distribution. Fecal coliform counts over 10 per gram is the standard for contamination. One in five of the Consumers Union samples had counts *exceeding 100 per gram!*

The American fish industry is a stinking mess. Preliminary results of the Food and Drug Administration's review of 3,852 fish-processing plants released in February 1992, were so bad that they formed the new Office of Seafood to try to regain control. Even so, they tell me that the problems will take years to solve.[2] If you are going to use fish as a low-fat source of protein, you have to protect yourself.

"Your flounder sir," the waiter said, placing before me a fishbone with eyeballs, attached to a bit of brown raincoat.
Michael Colgan

Finding Good Fish

Fresh fish has virtually no smell. As soon as it starts to go bad, fish produces a chemical called **tri-methylamine** which gives it the fishy odor. It's a definite sign of spoilage. The first rule in buying fish is: if it smells fishy, don't.

The next rule is to avoid certain fish altogether. Avoid swordfish (mercury and PCB contamination), lake whitefish (PCB contamination), oysters, mussels and clams (lead contamination), the large tuna species, yellowfin and bigeye (mercury contamination).

Many ocean and lake areas are so badly contaminated that the fish from them are deliberately mislabeled so you don't know where they come from. But, if you can find out, don't buy Great Lakes fish, fish from the Los Angeles Basin, the San Francisco Basin, the New Jersey coast, Puget Sound, and the Boston Harbor area. The Environmental Protection Agency, and numerous other studies report that all are heavily contaminated.[3]

A few more don'ts:

- Don't buy from stores that display cooked and raw fish on the same layer of ice, even if they are separated.

- Don't buy from stores that pile fish so high that the top fillets get heated by the case lights.

- Never buy a whole fish unless it is completely embedded in ice, has bright bulging eyes, and vivid color.

Buy the fish from Alaska, Australia and New Zealand, whose waters are low in pollutants. Unfortunately, even some Alaskan fish are now threatened by leaking radioactive wastes from defunct Soviet testing sites on the islands of Novaya Zwmlya, and from widespread radioactivity in runoff of the Ob and Yenisey rivers in Siberia.[4] So if that Alaska or Arctic salmon glows in the dark - bury it.

I have not discussed Scandinavian fish because trade restrictions make most of it history. That "fresh Norwegian salmon" usually isn't. For poor man's salmon, buy only the small species of tuna, skipjack, and albacore. Being lower on the food chain, they are only lightly polluted. Buy flounder and sole, the least polluted fish in the Consumer Union Study. Buy Australasian orange roughy: extremely low-fat and virtually contamination free.

Canned tuna, the most popular fish in America, deserves the last word. There is no bacteria problem because the canning involves high heat that kills everything. But, tests by the Consumers Union showed that 50% of the cans they bought contained filth from insects, rodents, and birds. In the early '70s there was a similar stink over canned fish. With a massive clean-up effort, tuna was cleaned of virtually all filth by 1979.[1] But since then, almost all canning has moved outside the U.S. to countries that have low-low standards of hygiene. So it will be a hard problem to fix.

Overall best tuna in the Consumers Union Study was canned albacore (white tuna). Best water-packed brands of albacore for taste and cost are Bumble Bee, Lady Lee and Empress Fancy. At less than one gram of fat per 100 grams (3½ oz), and 24 grams of first-class protein, tuna is still one of your best choices.

The best tuna I have found is from a small California company: unbleached albacore, hand caught (not net caught), and with no oil, water or salt added. Dave's Albacore is *the* tuna to eat. You can get it by calling (408)479-0211.

Chapter 7

Pesticides in Produce

With traditional methods of soil enrichment, plants obtain the minerals and other substances required to make natural chemical compounds in their leaves, stems and roots that discourage insects from eating them. This system worked pretty well for thousands of years.

But plants grown in mineral depleted soils, supported only by NPK fertilizers, no longer get enough of the nutrients required to produce their insect repellent compounds. They become easy prey to pests. Consequently, as use of NPK fertilizers spread throughout America, it became necessary to protect the weakened crops they grow, against pests that were previously controlled by traditional farming methods. So developed the new business empire of pesticides to further damage and poison our food.

In her great book **Silent Spring**, Rachel Carson reported that, by 1947, America was deluging crops with 120 million pounds of highly toxic chemicals. She showed conclusively how we were poisoning the land.[1] In that same year, Congress passed the first Federal Insecticide, Fungicide and Rodenticide Act. It required only that pesticide manufacturers register their products and label them with warnings to prevent farm workers from being poisoned.[2] No regulations prevented these poisons from entering our food, water, and air.

Rachel Carson was vilified by the corrupt chemical interests of the day and their political henchmen. They used every scurrilous trick in the book to discredit her work, and prevent the public from learning the truth. Fortunately, they could not prevent history from proving her right.

It took another 15 years of overwhelming evidence, that pesticides were causing cancer and other diseases in the general population, before government accepted that agribusiness greed had poisoned the American food chain from soil to table. In 1972, Congress passed a new act to protect our food, water and air, and created the Environmental Protection Agency (EPA) to enforce it.[3]

Since then, despite the regulations, we have suffered two decades of the most inept, corrupt, and impotent enforcement it is possible to imagine. Today 2.6 billion pounds of pesticides are spread on America every year.[4] That's 10 pounds for you, 10 pounds for me, 10 pounds for every breathing one of us.

DDT for example, was banned in 1972, but use of stocks and illegal use continued unchecked. By the late 1970s, there was so much DDT in mothers' milk in America, that it would have been illegal to carry it across state lines in any other container.

Currently used toxic pesticides include **captan, alachlor, 1,3-dichloropropene, dinoseb, ethyl dibromide, lindane, pronamide** and **trifluralin**. I have singled these out, because all of them have been cited as probable human carcinogens by the EPA's own special review process.[5] That is, repeated controlled experimental studies have shown conclusively that these chemicals cause cancer.

Yet, because of ineffective enforcement, all continue in use, along with 600 other toxic chemicals that form the basis of the more than 50,000 pesticide products used in America today.[6] Recent tests by the FDA of 26 fruits and vegetables, found residues of these products in 9,600 out of 20,000 samples.[7] So there is about a 50/50 chance that the apple pie you had for lunch, or the carrots you had for dinner, are contaminated.

"How could this happen?", cry indignant members of my lecture audiences.

I answer, "The same way the S & L disaster happened, ineffective government, arrogance and greed."

If you value your health, you will start today to buy only certified organic grains, breads, vegetables and fruits, and fish from unpolluted waters, such as the seas around Australia and New Zealand. If you don't you are courting disease. The types of disease and the risks you take with faulty nutrition, we cover in Chapters 11-13.

Chapter 8

Water, Water Everywhere . . .

Three-quarters of President Clinton's brain is water. So is yours. Every creature in Creation is mostly water. Your muscles are 70% water. Your blood is 82% water. Even your bones are a quarter water. This basic biochemistry emphasizes that *the most important component of your body is plain H$_2$0*.

The quality of your muscles, bones, organs and brain, their biochemistry, their resistance to injury and disease, and their longevity, is absolutely dependent on the purity of the water that you drink. As we head for health-care reform, let's hope that Mr. Clinton's brain is thinking with clean water.

Most Americans are not. Despite multiple warnings, the majority still use faucet water to drink and cook. Don't be one of them. Almost all faucet water in America today comes from polluted sources.[1] In 1988 the US Department of Public Health warned that 85% of American drinking water is contaminated.

Today, 7 July 1994, we tested the San Diego city water as it came out of our office faucet. The water authority claims it is clean, but the test showed 595 parts per million contaminants. That's about average. Some city waters are a bit cleaner, others a lot dirtier. You should not be drinking any of them.

The problems are multiple and completely out of control. Almost all the ground water in America is now contaminated with man-made chemicals. More than 55,000 of the *regulated* chemical dumps are leaking into the water table.[2]

Even at super-controlled Los Alamos, with every regulation and control system known to man, radioactive wastes have migrated into the ground water for miles around the dump.[3] Imagine the state of the estimated 200,000 illegal, *unregulated* chemical dumps in America leaking into the water table all across the nation.

Then there's bacteria. We look askance at South American water because of "tourista" and other water-borne infections. But our own is nearly as bad. Government figures show that over 900,000 people become ill each year from drinking US water laced with bacterial disease.[4]

> The hitherandthithering waters
> gather man's poisons
> from the land.
>
> *Michael Colgan*
> *Nutrition Lectures, 1994*

Not A Drop To Drink

But they clean the water don't they? No! Water treatment authorities treat water to minimum standards. More than 60,000 different chemicals now contaminate our water supplies. It's incredibly difficult and expensive to get them out with the obsolete and under-funded treatment systems now in use. The Natural Resources Defense Council has just reported that over two-thirds of our water treatment plants are obsolete.[5]

Water engineers are loathe to admit these problems. They do what they can with the resources available. The average water treatment station can afford to test for only 30-40 chemicals, and then try to remove about half that number. The other 59,980 chemicals have free rein to assault your body.

Even those they do try to remove often remain. Lead, for example, was finally banned from water in 1986 by The Safe Drinking Water Amendment Act. But the Environmental Protection Agency's latest report in 1993, shows that 819 water systems throughout America have toxic levels of lead remaining in the fully treated water.[6]

Even lead is the least of our water worries. Most drinking water supplies carry multiple toxins. In an overall test of 954 cities, the Office of Technology Assessment, the watchdog arm of Congress, reports that the drinking water of almost one-third of them is "seriously contaminated".[7]

Water authorities also *add* toxic chemicals such as chlorine and aluminum to water, chemicals that have no place in your body. Chlorination is an obsolete method for preventing epidemics of disease. But from the getgo 50 years ago, scientists knew it was toxic.

The chlorine reacts with organic wastes, which incidentally are left in the water, to form **trihalomethanes.** Trihalomethanes are known carcinogens that increase the risk of colon and rectal cancer, and *double* the risk of bladder cancer. Bladder cancer now strikes 40,000 Americans every year.[8,9,10] You don't want to join that crowd.

Finding Clean Water

I hope the evidence convinces you to get clean water. But *caveat emptor.* Bottled water is booming with over 500 brands on the market. Most of them are simply faucet water passed through "conditioning filters" to make it taste good and sell expensive.[11] The new labelling laws will *eventually* restrict the use of "spring", "mineral", and other buzz words. But the only bottled water likely to be clean is distilled water. Seven brands we have tested show 2-12 parts per million contaminants. That's about as clean as you can get.

Don't believe the hogwash put out by "spring" and "mineral" water companies that distilled water leaches the minerals from your body by osmotic pressure or similar tomfoolery. Any basic college text will reassure you that the human system doesn't work that way. If it did, your cells would be at the mercy of all the varying osmotic gradients created in your gut by every meal you eat.

Another bogus argument is that distilled water doesn't provide essential minerals. Neither do "mineral waters", at least in any useful quantity. We get our minerals mainly from vegetables or from supplements made directly from mineral-rich soils. As world authority on minerals, Dr. Eric Underwood says, "Plant materials provide the main source of minerals to most members of the human race".[12]

A good alternative to bottled distilled water is a decent home distiller, or a multiple-filter reverse osmosis system. But, again, *caveat emptor*. Every con man and his brother are selling water filters, swearing that they are FDA or EPA approved, and that they produce water of such cleanliness it is right next to Godliness.

Neither Government departments nor the Almighty approve water filters, because most of them just don't work. Before you buy, insist on a water purification test, comparing your tap water with the same tap water after it has been through the filter. If the finished product is more than 30 ppm contaminants, show the carpetbagger and his snakeoil gadget the door.

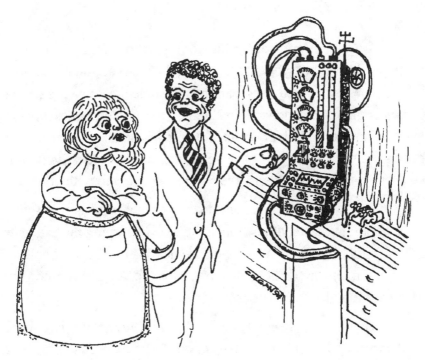

"You'll be amazed how the little Water Beauty simplifies your life."

Chapter 9

Degraded Food Degrades You

To obtain optimal health from nutrition, first you need to grasp just how much you affect your body by what you put in your mouth. The human body was carefully designed to convert a mix of certain compounds that occur in Nature into muscles, bones, organs, glands, and brain. The hairy bags of chemical soup that we call human beings *are* the interactions of these nutrient compounds. Every time you screw around with them, they will screw around with you.

Folk who scarf down fat-loaded burgers and nutrient-poor fries, do not understand how much they are disturbing the exquisite precision of nutrient use by their bodies. Let's use a couple of examples to illustrate how that precision makes the engine of a Masserati look like a child's toy.

Vitamin B_{12} is a good one. You require only a few micrograms (millionths of a gram) of B_{12} each day: the RDA is only 2 micrograms.[1] Your blood contains only about 5 nanograms (billionths of a gram) per liter, less than a speck of dust. You couldn't see that amount even under a microscope. It represents less than one part per trillion of your bodyweight. Yet if you lack that infintesimal speck, your whole body declines into the serious disease of pernicious anemia, which gradually destroys the myelin sheaths protecting your nerves, leading to blindness, insanity, and death.[2]

A second example is iodine. About 50 micrograms per day is considered sufficient for most people.[1] This is still an amount so tiny you could hardly see it on the head of a pin. Every day your body separates out the few molecules of iodine that occur in different foods with a precision far beyond the most advanced computer, and transports them straight to the thyroid gland. There they convert an inert chemical called thyronine into powerful thyroid hormones. These hormones then control your energy supply, your mood, and even how well you can think.[3]

The same applies to other micronutrients. It is still a mystery to science how such minute amounts of these substances can hold the keys to health, to sanity, even to life itself. But they do, and if they are deficient in your food, you are asking for disease.

Your health at 80 is a profit or a loss on the investment you make in health today.
Michael Colgan
Nutrition Lectures, 1994

Essential Nutrients

Optimal bodily function cannot occur without daily ingestion of a precise mix of the 59 nutrients shown in Table 3. Some you need a lot of, others, you need only tiny amounts. But they all have to be provided in the *correct* amounts. The first five, **oxygen, hydrogen, carbon, nitrogen, and sulfur,** you need in large amounts. They are widely dispersed in foods and in the air you breathe, so supply is not often a problem. The remaining 54 nutrients you need in medium or small amounts, but they are less plentiful in the environment. More important, they may be deficient or entirely absent in many of the degraded foods that now form most of the American food supply.

We know that 13 vitamins, 22 minerals, 6 co-factors (helper substances), 8 amino acids (plus 3 more in certain circumstances), and 2 essential fatty acids are required for optimal bodily function. All these essential substances interact with each other in precise synergy to produce, maintain, and renew your body. If even one is missing, or in short supply, then the functions of all the others are impaired.[4]

Although the essentiality of co-factors is still controversial, I have included them, because recent evidence all points in that direction. In science jargon, the word "essential" means:

(a)The nutrients have to be present in adequate amounts or function is impaired.

(b) the body cannot make the nutrients or cannot make enough of them for normal tissue function.

(c) you have to get them from your diet.

**Table 3: Vitamins and co-factors, essential elements, essential
fatty acids and amino acids required for the human body.**

Elements required in large amounts daily:

Oxygen	Hydrogen	Nitrogen
Carbon	Sulfur	

Elements required in medium amounts daily:

Calcium	Magnesium	Potassium
Phosphorus	Sodium	Chloride

Elements required in small amounts daily:

Iron	Zinc	Copper
Manganese	Silicon	Cobalt
Chromium	Selenium	Iodine
Fluoride	Molybdenum	Nickel
Arsenic	Boron	Tin*
Germanium*	*Probable essential elements*	

Vitamins (common form names):

A (retinol)	B1 (thiamin)	B2 (riboflavin)
B3 (niacin, niacinamide)	B5 (pantothenic acid)	B6 (pyridoxine)
B12 (cobalamin)	Folic acid	Biotin
C (ascorbic acid)	D (calciferol)	E (d-alpha tocopherol)
K (phylloquinone)		

Co-factors (common form names):

Choline	Inositol	Bioflavonoids
Para-amino-benzoic acid (PABA)		Co-enzyme Q10
Pyroloquinoline quinone (PQQ)		

Essential amino acids:

Isoleucine	Leucine	Lysine
Methionine	Phenylalanine	Threonine
Tryptophan	Valine	Arginine‡
Histidine‡	Taurine‡	*‡ Conditionally essential*

Essential fatty acids:

Linoleic acid	Linolenic acid

Sources: Colgan Institute, San Diego, CA., & References 1 and 3.

We Are Deficient

Let us look now at some of the official government figures to see how the degraded foods that most people eat do not provide sufficient nutrients. **The Health and Nutrition Examination Survey (HANES 1)** studied 28,000 people, from age 1 to 74, in sixty-five different areas throughout the United States.[5] **HANES 1** examined the diets people actually ate, the levels of nutrients in their blood, and any symptoms of malnutrition. Using very conservative levels as the norm, it found huge dietary deficiencies.

For instance, nine women out of every ten had insufficient iron in their diets (less than 18 mg). One in every two women had insufficient calcium (less than 600 mg). Iron deficiency in the blood was widespread in all age, sex, race and income groups, despite the fact that white bread and cereals in America are "enriched" with iron. Overall, more than 60% of these people showed at least one symptom of malnutrition, regardless of their income level.

The **Ten State Nutritional Survey** of 86,000 people found similar evidence.[6] In Michigan for example, more than half the men and women tested were deficient in folic acid. In Texas and Washington one in every four men and one in every three women were deficient in Vitamin A. One in three persons in Southern California was deficient in Vitamin B_2 (riboflavin).

And these figures took the very conservative values of the RDAs as representing adequate nutrition. Nevertheless, about two-thirds of these people were malnourished even though the number of nutrients tested for deficiency was only a fifth of the 59 nutrients essential for optimal health.

A third government study showed similar results. **The**

Nationwide Food Consumption Survey of 15,000 households found that one household in three ate diets deficient in calcium and vitamin B6. One household in five ate diets deficient in iron and vitamin A.[7]

A recent report from the USDA examined another 37,785 people. It analyzed intakes of only 11 of the essential nutrients. Results showed that the vast majority of subjects ate less than the RDA of vitamins A and B6 and minerals, calcium, iron and magnesium.[8] The percentages of people in the study who were getting insufficient nutrients are shown in Table 4.

It gets worse as you get older. A new study of older Americans by Dr. Jacob Selhub and colleagues at the USDA Human Nutrition Research Center at Tufts University, examined diet and blood levels of just three nutrients, folate, B6 and B12. They found that 60% of these seniors got insufficient folate to prevent high levels of homocysteine in their blood, a proven risk factor for heart disease. The worst finding was that 80% of subjects were getting the RDA for folate, but that level of intake was clearly insufficient to keep them healthy.[9]

In an accompanying editorial to the study, published in the very conservative **Journal of the American Medical Association**, Professors Meir Stampfer and Walter Willett of Harvard University concluded, "a reasonable argument can be made for recommending . . . . . multi-vitamins for many individuals".[9]

Table 4: Nutrient Intake of Sample of 37,785 U.S. Citizens

Nutrient	% receiving less than the full RDA	% receiving the full RDA or more
Pyridoxine (B6)	80	20
Magnesium	75	25
Calcium	68	32
Iron	57	43
Vitamin A	50	50
Thiamin (B1)	45	55
Vitamin C	41	59
Riboflavin (B2)	34	66
Cobalamin (B12)	34	66
Niacin (B3)	33	67
Phosphorus	27	73

Source: United States Department of Agriculture, **Food Technology** 1981;35:9.

There are many other studies with similar results, but I will not bore you rigid with endless examples. The evidence we have reviewed is sufficient. It shows without a doubt, that average people eating the average degraded American food are seriously deficient in essential nutrients.

Hundreds of thousands of people have now realized these problems with our food, hence the burgeoning movement to return to organic farming. Sadly, it will take decades before even a quarter of American agricultural land is detoxified and then restored by years of mulching, manuring and crop rotation, to regain the nutrient-rich soils of our forefathers. Meanwhile you have to protect yourself. As we will see, you can restore your personal nutrient levels by using the right vitamin and mineral supplements. But before you can determine what supplements you need, I have to answer two questions:

> 1. Which nutrient deficiencies produce which diseases?

> 2. How much of each nutrient do you need for effective protection?

The following chapters provide that vital information.

One packaged food in every four charges you more for the container than the contents.
Tufts University Newsletter
August 1987

Chapter 10

Failure Of American Medicine

Health authorities keep telling us that we have never been healthier. The National Cancer Institute constantly claims that the cancer picture is improving. The Heart, Lung and Blood Institute and the American Heart Association constantly claim that their work is responsible for the decline in cardiovascular disease since 1970. The FDA constantly claims that it is effectively protecting the nation's health. As we see in this and the next three chapters, *they are all lying through their teeth.*

Physicians and health bureaucrats in almost every medical speciality you can name, attend my lectures. Afterwards, some of them buttonhole me or send me long and indignant letters describing advances in medical technology, or development of wonder drugs that have improved the treatment of major diseases. On the surface their reasoning sounds impeccable, but it is mostly dead wrong.

New drugs and medical gizmos may appear to work in the clinical trials that get them FDA approval. But the only real test of their effectiveness, is whether or not they reduce morbidity (disability) or mortality in the general population.

We can argue interminably about morbidity. Is it an advance for example, to be able to do atheroscopic surgery for a torn cartilage in your knee, through a tiny hole instead of by open surgery. It seems so for many reasons, including less surgical trauma, less healing time, greatly reduced risk of infection, etc. But then you read the controlled studies, showing that people with torn cartilages who opt not to have surgery at all, have better healing, less pain, and less arthritic degeneration of the knee in later life.[1]

So I am not going to look at morbidity. The only medical measurement about which there is no argument is mortality.

Death Tells The Truth

I like death, as a measurement that is. Death is so nice and final. After a day or two of decay, even the most stubborn physician has to agree that the treatment just isn't working.

With every medical speciality claiming great advances, then there should be less death. When we cut through all the statistical nonsense about treatments, good health care yields longer life, bad health care yields shorter life. Period!

Let's see how America stacks up. Table 5 shows the latest official figures comparing life expectancy at birth for males and females for all major countries in Western Europe and the Mediterranean, plus Canada, Australia, Japan, and the US. Out of 21 countries, America ranks 18th!

How can this be? Britain and Japan spend only 6% of their Gross National Product on health care. We spend over 12%,[2] and have every medical widget known to man. Surely we should be top of the list. But we're not.

The grim fact is that *the health care system claimed by President Clinton to be, "the best anywhere", is actually near the worst.* Compared with the Japanese, who spend less than half of what we do on health care, Table 5 shows that the American system chops 4 years off the average life span for females and 3 years for males.[3] That's the bad news, and its getting worse by the year.

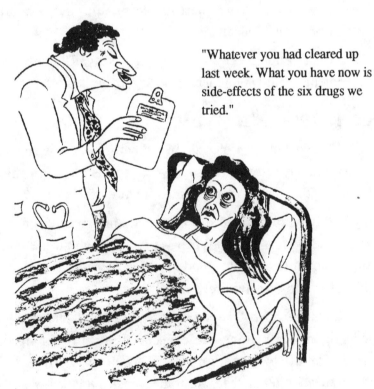

"Whatever you had cleared up last week. What you have now is side-effects of the six drugs we tried."

Table 5: Life Expectancy at birth for selected developed countries 1990, listed best to worst.

Region/Country	Male	Female
Japan	76.4	82.1
Switzerland	75.2	82.6
Spain	74.8	81.6
Italy	74.5	81.4
Sweden	74.7	80.7
Netherlands	74.2	81.1
France	73.4	81.9
Greece	75.0	80.2
Canada	74.0	80.7
Norway	73.3	80.8
Germany	73.4	80.6
Austria	73.5	80.4
Belgium	73.4	80.4
Australia	73.5	79.8
England/Wales	73.3	79.2
Denmark	72.6	78.8
United States	**72.1**	**79.0**
New Zealand	72.2	78.4
Finland	71.1	79.9
Portugal	70.9	78.0

Source: Kinsella KG. 1992 (Reference 3)

Medicine For Profit

Our health care used to be good. How do I know? Again, death is the most reliable statistic. Let's look at life expectancy figures again, this time for 1950. Table 6 shows that America ranked 7th, eleven solid places further up the list than where it is now.

For the last 40 years our health care has gone downhill. As the table shows, in 1950 we were way ahead of advanced countries like Switzerland, Japan, and Canada. Now we are way behind.

How did our health care fail? Corruption and greed folks, corruption and greed. Harvard scientist Dr. Paul Starr explains in his elegant book, **The Social Transformation of American Medicine**.[4] After the Second World War, medicine in America started to become an industry rather than a profession. By the '50s, the giant pharmaceutical companies, the hospital companies, the ambulance companies, the medical equipment companies, wrested the control of medicine out of the hands of the physicians, and put it into the hands of entrepreneurs. Medicine for profit rather than health began.

This social disaster forged ahead in earnest in 1968, when the Humana organization began buying hospitals and setting up a much-copied, high-profit, cookie-cutter model of health care to be provided throughout its holdings. Physicians, administrators, and hospital service organizations all had to toe the corporate line.

How much profit? If you bought a share of Humana in 1968, it cost $8. By 1980, 12 years later, it was worth $336 - an increase of 4200%.[4] That's an obscene amount of money extracted from human suffering.

Table 6: Life Expectancy at birth for selected developed countries 1950, listed best to worst.

Region/Country	Male	Female
Norway	70.3	73.8
Netherlands	70.3	72.6
Sweden	69.9	72.6
Denmark	68.9	71.5
New Zealand	67.2	71.3
Australia	66.7	71.8
United States	**66.0**	**71.7**
Canada	66.4	70.9
England/Wales	66.2	71.1
Switzerland	66.4	70.8
Germany	64.6	68.5
France	63.7	69.4
Italy	63.7	67.2
Greece	63.4	66.7
Belgium	62.1	67.4
Austria	62.0	67.0
Finland	61.1	67.9
Spain	59.8	64.3
Japan	59.6	63.1
Portugal	55.6	60.7

Source: Kinsella KG. 1992 (Reference 3)

Humana is only one example of profits from illness that make nonsense of current government and media bleatings that health care is a basic right. Government controlled hospitals now total less than 5% of available hospital beds in America. Current US health care is simply business as usual, an industry, that over the last 40 years, has proved itself to be supremely ineffective in maintaining the nation's health. If you want to remain fit and strong, stay as far away from it as you can for as long as you can.

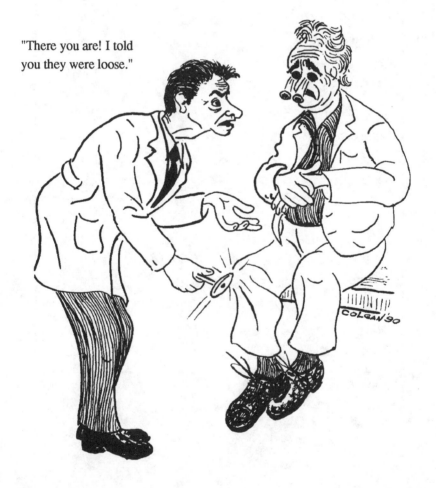

"There you are! I told you they were loose."

Chapter 11

Heart Disease: Man-made Plague

Despite media hyperbole, the worst killers in America are not AIDS, or traffic accidents, or disenfranchised youths with automatic weapons. The grim reaper's most destructive troops are the chronic degenerative diseases with long incubation periods. For decades they grow silently inside you, only to emerge in a time of stress, usually full-blown and incurable.

These modern-day monsters are cardiovascular diseases, cancers, adult-onset diabetes, lung diseases and liver diseases. They are our top five causes of pain, suffering, and premature death.[1]

The worst of it is, *all these diseases are predominantly man-made*. Let's look at our biggest killer - cardiovascular disease. With over one million premature deaths per year, it's hard to believe we caused it all ourselves. But we did.

The Rise Of Coronary Disease

The first report of coronary artery disease in America was published in 1912 in the **Journal of the American Medical Association** by Dr. James Herrick.[2] The disease was so rare that famous cardiologist, Dr. Paul Dudley White, spent the next 10 years searching for it and found only three cases.[3] Today we have thousands of cases in any small city.

In the same medical journal 77 years later, on July 7 1989, a nationwide analysis showed that 60 million American adults aged 20-90, now have coronary disease to some degree.[4] There is no longer any doubt that the wanton destruction of our food, air, and water, and the inept and corrupt work of our health authorities created this monster, and it is alive and growing in every third one of us.

Humbug physicians will object that cardiovascular disease is declining, because modern medicine has become so wonderful at detecting it early and treating it successfully. *Don't believe them!* Even advanced cardiovascular disease is very difficult to detect. The excruciating first symptom as the monster awakes, is often the only one you ever feel, a few hours before it kills you.

Dr. Lewis Kuller, for example, analyzed records of 326 people who died of sudden heart attacks, all of whom had received medical examinations within six months before death. Eighty-six of the subjects had received medical examinations within the seven days before their death. *Not a single one of the heart attacks had been predicted by their physicians.*[5]

Medical Treatment Poor at Cure

If you are fortunate enough to have cardiovascular disease correctly diagnosed before it manifests as a heart attack or stroke, then surely modern treatment can tackle it? No way! Most medical therapies for cardiovascular disease are simply symptomatic relief, that does nothing to reverse or even to arrest the disease process.

How can I make such an outrageous statement against all the TV portrayals of heart transplants, quadruple bypasses, and other marvels, performed by heroic medicos fighting to fit their simian fingers to vast machines, whose syncopated chirps and robotic responses rival R2D2 from Star Wars, and seem more than capable of breathing life into an ailing garden gnome? Easy. Unlike television, I have no market share or advertisers to satisfy, so I can tell you the truth.

It's tough to find evidence for or against the efficacy of American medical treatment, because usually there is nothing to compare it with. One valid comparison we can make is between the US and Canada, countries that have similar lifestyles and rates of cardiovascular disease. Canadian socialized medicine does not pay for the extensive treatments, surgeries, and lavish rehabilitation programs used routinely in the US. Treatment there for cardiovascular disease is often limited to inexpensive dietary and lifestyle manipulations, together with supporting medication. Here we routinely perform coronary arteriography, angioplasty, revascularization, and 170,000 bypass operations a year.

Despite all this high-tech, horrendously expensive treatment, a recent comparison of similar patients in the US and Canada showed ***no difference at all in mortality rates*** or the rate of second heart attacks.[6] Our health-care for cardiovascular disease works about as well on patients as it does on garden gnomes.

Bypasses: No Advance

Let's look at that bastion of heart savers, the bypass operation. As I write, the news wires are humming with reports that movie star Tony Curtis had a double bypass yesterday. Even the advisors of the rich and famous are convinced that it works. Then there's the TV portrayals. With fantastic skill, surgeons graft on new blood vessels to feed the heart, by detouring around the blocked coronary arteries. Meanwhile, amazing heart-lung machines breathe for the patient, clean his blood, keep the blood pumping and perform dozens of other life-sustaining tasks. Surely such advanced electronic wizardry has to work better than the 100-year-old traditional advice to cut the fat in your diet and go for a daily walk?

The government Coronary Artery Surgery Study spent 24 million dollars of your tax money to find out. Their study examined records of 16,626 angiogram patients. From these records, researchers selected 780 patients with good heart function, but a significant blockage of one or more coronary arteries. Half the patients were given bypass surgery plus drugs. The other half were treated with nutritional and lifestyle changes plus drugs. *Bypass surgery conferred no advantage at all, neither in longevity nor in incidence of future heart attacks.*[7]

> It's only logical that anyone who believes in American medicine should also believe in faith healing.
>
> *Michael Colgan*
> *Medical Lectures, 1994*

Don't Do Drugs

What if you avoid surgery and just use our wonderful new drugs instead? I wouldn't. The **Johns Hopkins Medical Letter** reports on fatal drug reactions in hospitals, where you would think medical expertise would protect you, or at least where they can save you if a drug reaction occurs. *Prescribed hospital drugs are so toxic they kill 130,000 Americans every year.*[8]

Outside the hospitals, the death toll from the same prescription drugs is probably a lot higher, but is frequently unreported or listed simply as heart failure. The **1994 Physicians Desk Reference** contains hundreds of pages of side-effects of common prescription drugs used for cardiovascular disease. Side effects include many kinds of cancer, heart disease, liver disease, brain damage, and sudden death.[9]

It isn't all corruption and greed. Many individual physicians are the finest of people, who do their best with our hopelessly flawed system of health care. But the record speaks for itself. I could go on throughout this whole book, citing study after study from my files, showing that once cardiovascular disease manifests, medicine can do little to help you.

Yet, as we saw above, this is mostly a man-made ailment, so we should be able to find what causes it and to avoid those risks. And we can. Do not fear cardiovascular disease. It is the easiest of all man-made diseases to prevent, and even to reverse, if only you follow the right nutrition, plus a little easy exercise to blow away the cobwebs. Chapters 20 and 25 tell you all you need to know.

Chapter 12

We Are Losing The War On Cancer

Cancer is our second biggest killer, and it's getting worse. In February 1994, a government research team led by Dr. Devra Davis of the US Department of Health and Human Services, published the latest cancer figures in the **Journal of the American Medical Association**. Males of the baby-boomer generation, now entering their 40s and 50s, have *three times* the cancer rate of their grandfathers.[1]

Non-smoking female baby-boomers also have more cancer than their grandmothers. And females who smoke today, have six times the cancer of their grandmothers.[1] *Overall, the study shows that cancer incidence is increasing for all ages in America.*

What do cancer authorities say to this evidence? Dr. Cary Presant, chairman of the California Division of the American Cancer

Society says, "Everyone eventually dies of something."[2] Clark Heath of the American Cancer Society says, "I really don't think the study changes our perspective on .... what causes cancer."[3] Such wise and caring leadership sure fills me with confidence.

Edward Sondik, deputy director of the National Cancer Institute's Division of Cancer Prevention, calls the evidence that smoking males have only 10% more smoking-related cancers than their grandfathers, "A major public health victory."[3] That's the sort of help you can expect from the cancer authorities. If you want to beat cancer, you have to protect yourself.

The huge increase in the incidence of cancer should be more than enough to convince you. The National Cancer Institute agrees that one American in every three living today will get cancer.[4] In the 1990s that means 1,000,000 new cases every year. If you don't protect yourself, then your chances of avoiding cancer are getting pretty slim. And once you develop this disease your chance of successful treatment is the flip of a crooked nickel.

What we have is a science of illness. What we need is a science of health.

René Dubos

Cancer Treatment Has Not Improved

In 1971, then President Nixon declared a knock-down, drag-out "war on cancer." Billions of your tax dollars were allocated, and every year since, the National Cancer Institute (NCI) has claimed great progress. As we hit the mid '90s, it is obvious that most of these claims are false. If you developed cancer in 1970, the overall chance of a cure was less than 50/50. Today, it is still less than 50/50.

What about the wonders of modern chemotherapy drugs touted almost daily in the media? Eminent medical biostatician Dr. Ulrich Abel, spent a year analysing the efficacy of all forms of chemotherapy against all types of epithelial cancers. Epithelial cancers encompass all common cancers and account for 80% of our cancer deaths.

Abel did not find many cures. Instead he found that most clinical trials report success when the therapy causes tumors to shrink. These are the reports used by the media. Unfortunately, Abel also found that tumor shrinkage by chemotherapy does not cure the cancers, a fact often obscured by researchers, and not realized by most of the media.

Most important, after meticulously reviewing thousands of studies, he found that *"there is no evidence for the majority of cancers that treatment with these drugs exerts any positive influence on survival or quality of life in patients with advanced disease."*[5] In the majority of cancers, by the time the disease shows itself, it is advanced.

The final nail in the cancer coffin comes from the oncologists who treat patients with chemotherapy. Abel cites poll after poll of cancer physicians, showing that many would refuse chemotherapy if they developed cancer themselves.[5]

Cancer Death Rate Increasing

What about chemotherapy, radiation and surgery combined. Sorry to have to tell you that these three approved treatments for cancer are little better than no treatment at all. Let's look at breast cancer. The increasing incidence of breast cancer, now makes it the third leading cause of cancer deaths in America.[6] Against this rising tide, and the public outcry, the National Cancer Institute claims to have made a big reduction in breast cancer mortality.

Their false reasoning goes like this. In the 1960s, the breast cancer survival rate was 60%. Today it is 75%. Therefore we have improved survival by 15%. Some ignorant national media have been easily manipulated to trumpet these figures as a great success.

The truth is more sobering. First, in order to justify their multi-billion dollar budgets, the cancer *industry,* I use the word deliberately, devised the term "survival" to replace "cure". "Survival" means that the person lives five years or longer after the cancer is diagnosed.

An investigation by the General Accounting Office, the watchdog arm of Congress, shows that breast cancer is now being diagnosed much earlier.[7] It is usually a slow-growing cancer that develops gradually for up to 20 years before it kills you. If more of the cases are being diagnosed at earlier stages of development, it's obvious that more will be alive five years later, *whether they are treated or not.*

The NCI claims of improvement have little to do with better treatments, and mostly to do with finding more cases of early breast cancer. In fact the NCI's own figures show that more young women are now dying of breast cancer than ever before.[6,7]

NCI figures show the same grim picture for cancer overall. In May 1986, in the **New England Journal of Medicine**, cancer experts Dr. John Bailor of Harvard and Dr. Eileen Smith of the University of Iowa, published a precise analysis of NCI figures, which showed unequivocally that overall cancer survival rates have not improved at all. On the contrary, *from 1950 to 1980 the cancer death rate in America steadily increased*.[8]

The increase in the cancer death rate, which means a *decline* in the cure rate, and which shows unequivocally that current medical treatment for cancer does not work, should convince you that the only answer is prevention. Don't fret. As I show in Chapters 19-21, you can provide your body with powerful weapons against cancer that are as easy to use, as straightforward, and as inexpensive as cleaning your teeth.

Do not fear cancer. As Professor Lewis Thomas, President of the Sloan Kettering Cancer Hospital tells us, the human body is incredibly tough. Given the right nutrition, exercise and lifestyle, it will resist cancer for a lifetime.

Chapter 13

Osteoporosis Is Epidemic

Lora McCarthy was 81 when she slipped and fell to the floor. A mild fall that would have a healthy person springing up in embarrassment. But it broke Lora's pelvis in three places. She is one of the 25 million of us who have osteoporosis, the weak and brittle bone disease.

Lora was lucky. She was treated by a smart physician who rejected drugs in favor of a program of superior nutrition and daily exercise. Her pelvis healed quickly, and all her bones became progressively stronger. The osteoporosis was reversed simply by giving her body the nutrients and activity that it needed. Now Lora travels widely and never misses her nutrient supplements and daily exercise.[1]

Margaret _____ was not so lucky. A gifted concert violinist, her 5'8" height and erect posture added grace to her performances. Until her early 50's that is, when osteoporosis began to show. Her spine curved in such a dowager's hump that her ribs came to rest on her pelvis. She could no longer play the violin.

No one advised her about optimal nutrition, nor about exercise. After years of pain and palliative drugs, she suffered a spontaneous hip fracture, deteriorated quickly and died. At death Margaret measured 4'-6".[2]

Which do you want to be, Lora or Margaret? The choice is all yours. Osteoporosis used to be uncommon. Now the **Harvard Medical School Newsletter** calls it "a silent epidemic".[3]

One in every two American women and one in every four American men over 50 are afflicted. They suffer more than 2,000,000 broken bones every year. With our degraded nutrition and sedentary lifestyle, we did it all to ourselves.

This book is too small to cover every man-made disease in detail. That would take twenty volumes. But because osteoporosis is so misunderstood, yet so simple to prevent, I would like to spell it out good.

Foods Affect Your Bones

Common foods have a big influence on your bones. Normal levels of protein for example, do not affect bone calcium,[4] but we know now that some forms of purified protein do cause calcium loss. Notably, casein, lactalbumin, and egg white, that are commonly used in meal replacement drinks, can seriously deplete your calcium stores, if they are used as the main source of protein in your diet.[5,6]

Very high protein intakes as used by many strength athletes, and by folk on those idiotic high protein diet plans, suck calcium out of your body like a sponge.[7] So these folk should always be aware of their unique need for increased calcium intake.[8]

Salt also robs your bones. Our diet is spiked with twenty times the salt that occurs in natural food, and that is twenty times the salt required for optimal health. This sodium overload inhibits normal calcium metabolism in complex ways, all of which are detrimental to a wide range of bodily functions including blood pressure and bone formation.[8a] So ditch the salt cellar and the chips.

Fiber doesn't help either. High intakes of fiber don't rob your bones, but they do inhibit calcium absorption from the intestines. So when you take fiber for good health, as you should, always be aware that it increases your need for calcium.[9]

What about vegetables? Numerous tables of calcium sources list spinach as one of the best, containing 120-150 mg of calcium per average serving. Wrong! Wrong! Wrong! We have known for 40 years that spinach also contains high levels of chemicals called **oxalates**, that completely bind the calcium so that not even a milligram can be absorbed.[10]

So spinach is useless. Much better are green cabbage, kale, broccoli, bok choy, dark green lettuces, and the seaweed greens, arame, hijiki and nori.

Other good food sources of calcium are salmon and sardines canned with bones, well-cooked soybeans, tofu, and soy milk. But most people don't get enough of them because, as we see in Chapter 16, the average calcium intake is way below the RDA of 800 - 1200 mg per day. And we know the lower RDA is insufficient for anyone. Dr. Herta Spencer has shown repeatedly that normal adults require at least 1200 mg of calcium per day to remain in calcium balance.[11]

Even if we did get sufficient calcium, it's only a tiny piece of the bone puzzle. There's a lot more to bone than stuffing your face with chalk.

Then There's Milk

For the last 40 years, the dominant medical advice, delivered with much pomp and pretension, has been: drink two large glasses of milk a day. That amount of milk contains 600 mg of calcium, and what could be more innocuous than milk - right? Wrong! For many folk, *the medical advice to drink milk to prevent osteoporosis is self-serving poppycock.*

How do I know? Simple. After four decades of milk promotion, osteoporosis has become epidemic. Milk just doesn't do the trick.

Animal milk was designed by the miraculous hand that guides Nature specifically for nourishing infant animals, not human adults. As we grow, we lose much of our ability to produce the enzyme **lactase**, which digests the lactose in milk. Three out of every four American adults have some degree of lactose intolerance.[12] Many folk with osteoporosis are so lactose-intolerant they can't touch dairy foods without severe discomfort.

It gets worse. Lactose-intolerant folk, especially women, should not drink milk anyway. Far from being the innocuous food it is for infants, there is now a pile of evidence that milk is toxic to adults. Dr. Daniel Cramer at Harvard Medical School for example, has shown that plain "wholesome" milk increases the risk of ovarian cancer in lactose-intolerant women. And he and other researchers have just published a meticulous analysis of lactose-intolerant women in 36 countries, and numerous human and animal studies, showing that **galactose**, a component sugar of lactose, is toxic to the ovaries, inhibits fertility, and may produce defective children.[13]

Of course you can use lactase pills to help, or you can drink lactose-free milk. But neither strategy is ideal. The lactase pills are very hit-and-miss, and removing the lactose from milk reduces the absorption of the calcium by as much as 50%.[14] So leave the milk for those it really benefits - baby MOOs.

Bones and Aging

Many physicians have a legitimate excuse for their ignorance of bone. As in the medical school I taught at, they were taught that bone mass declines as a direct consequence of aging. The usual table shows increasing bone mass until age 30-35, then bone losses of about 1% per year until death, with accelerated bone loss of 5-8% per year in women after menopause.[15] *This belief, that you cannot help losing your bones to the passing years, is completely false.*

Nevertheless, many people, including physicians, accept the figures, because they are based on careful and repeated studies of representative samples of average Americans. But, as we have seen, average Americans are undernourished, overweight, and sedentary. So measurement of the bones of samples of these people presents a completely false picture of the bones of optimally nourished, active folk.

There is an important lesson here, ignorance of which has led American medicine into multiple errors. Science can never discover the optimal state, or even the normal state, of the human body by measuring Mr. & Mrs. Average. From such measurements, we used to believe that blood pressure and cholesterol rise with age, that middle-age spread is inevitable, that strength declines with age, and that sexuality disappears altogether. These and a host of other apparent markers of aging have now proved to be false.

World expert on aging Dr. John Rowe of Harvard Medical School puts it best, "The detrimental changes that occur with age in representative samples of the population create a false gerontology, a gerontology of the usual".[16]

So you can safely discard all notions of inevitable bone loss with age, and focus instead on the strategies that grow strong bones and keep them strong lifelong.

Growing Strong Bones

Obsolete medical teaching states that all you need to do for strong bones is eat sufficient calcium. Pharmaceutical companies and the dairy industry have spent many $$ millions maintaining this story in the hearts and minds of America, because it sells $$ billions worth of calcium pills and dairy products every year. Americans now consume enough calcium pills to solidify the entire House of Representatives, yet osteoporosis grows steadily worse.

In condoning this enterprise, the FDA must have access to superior knowledge than mere science, because the scientific evidence shows unequivocally that, by themselves, *calcium supplements just don't work*.[17,18]

The reason they don't work is simple:- *synergy*. Supplementing with any *single* nutrient cannot possibly work in the mind-boggling complexity of that biochemical soup we call human beings. Nutrients work only by interaction with other nutrients.

For optimal interaction, all the nutrients involved in a particular process have to be present in amounts that balance each other. If you put in a large excess of one nutrient such as calcium, over a period of months you may see a small increase in bone density. But it will not be a normal or healthy increase. You will also see an increase in calcium plaque in arteries, pathological calcification of soft tissues, and a large increase in urinary calcium.[19]

The body is dealing with the calcium excess by dumping it anywhere it can, so as to bring blood calcium levels back into workable ratios with the levels of other minerals. Once you realize the complex synergy of nutrients required to build bone, you will never again be tempted to take calcium supplements, nor supplements of any single nutrient.

Even the conservative U.S. National Academy of Sciences, states that normal bone formation requires calcium, vitamin D, zinc, copper, manganese, fluoride (more correctly, fluorine), silica (more correctly, silicon), and boron.[20] As I note throughout this book, most of these nutrients are deficient in American food and people. So if you are going to supplement with calcium it's only logical to supplement with other bone-forming nutrients also.

In addition, we have known for thirty years that the essential mineral magnesium acts to increase calcium absorption from the diet, and calcium retention in bone.[21] And new studies by Dr. Robert Neilsen and colleagues at the USDA Human Nutrition Research Center in Grand Forks, ND, show that without adequate magnesium, you lose bone like crazy.[22]

Recent studies also show that one in every four post-menopausal women can't absorb sufficient calcium to maintain bone, even at supplement levels of 1500 mg per day.[23] Dr. Guy Abrahams and colleagues show that if you add 600 mg of magnesium per day, then only 500 mg of calcium is required to cause a rapid increase in bone density, even in advanced osteoporosis.[24]

Supplementing with all the above minerals, plus vitamin D,

is still not enough for strong bones. Vitamin C for example, improves calcium absorption by up to 100%.[25] We now suspect that calcium interacts with most of the other 58 essential nutrients that compose the human body. New studies show that supplements of multiple vitamins and minerals, yield much greater increases in bone density than calcium, or calcium and vitamin D.[26] And the greater the number of the essential nutrients you add to the mix, the better the result.

This evidence is just one more piece of the puzzle showing that **complete nutrition** with all nutrients every day, which permits all essential nutrient interactions to take place, is the only road to optimum health. With the multiple nutrient deficiencies that government and medical authorities have allowed to creep into our food, it's no wonder America is losing its bones.

Lifestyle Destroys Bones

Even complete nutrition is still only half the bone story. Unhealthy lifestyles cause at least as much of our man-made osteoporosis as does faulty food. Let's look at a few of the biggies. Moderate intakes of alcohol, up to 2-3 drinks per day, do not affect your bones. But excess alcohol turns them into noodles. Even young alcoholics show severe bone loss.[27]

Another effect of alcohol is to turn your body acid. But our high-fat, high-sugar diet is far worse in creating acidity. So many Americans are now chronically acidic, that we spend $600 million on antacids every year.[28] Acidosis destroys your bones, because the body has to steal alkalizing minerals from them, to keep the blood Ph from dropping into the acid range where it starts to burn your cells.

There is an even more sinister twist. Leading antacids such as Maalox, Mylanta Gelusil, and Amphojel contain aluminum.

Numerous studies now show that even small amounts of aluminum antacids cause extensive bone loss. They deplete body phosphorus, and disrupt the essential calcium/phosphorus interactions that maintain bone.[29,30] Dr. Robert Heaney, osteoporosis specialist at Creighton University, Omaha, Nebraska, refers to this bodily pollution as "internal acid rain".

Far better to change your diet to less acid foods, and eliminate both acidity and the need to take antacids. It's simple. The Colgan Institute provides all clients with the list of acid and alkaline foods shown in Table 7. Use it for good health.

Other common and often unnecessary drugs that cause bone loss include cortisone, prednisone, and other glucocorticoids, thyroid hormones, barbiturate anticonvulsants, heparin, methotrexate, and cholestyramine.[31] If you take any of these, ask your physician about alternatives, or stopping altogether.

Exercise Your Bones

The biggest lifestyle problem in America today is couch potatoism. It's deadly to your bones. Bones are constantly remodelled throughout life in exact response to the stresses placed on them by activity. But not any old activity will do. Every day millions of old bone cells die off. In order to form new replacement cells, bone requires weight-bearing stress on each microscopic point where fibers of the bone matrix join together, much like the zig-zag connections of the girders of a bridge. Pressure on these stress points causes the essential electrochemical "sparks" that stimulate growth of new bone cells. No pressure, no sparks, no bone.

Common medical treatments illustrate only too well how lack of weight-bearing exercise destroys bone. We have known since the

Table 7: Effects of common foods on the body's acid/alkaline balance.

Acid Foods Avoid These	Neutral Foods Eat These	Alkaline Foods Always Eat These
All antibiotics	Apples	Baking soda
All fried foods	Apricots	Blackberries
Artificial sweeteners	Bananas	Broccoli
Beef	Beans - fresh & dried	Cantaloupe
Beer	Blueberries	Cinnamon
Butter	Buckwheat	Diakon radish
Carob	Cauliflower	Endive
Casein	Carrots	Garlic
Cheese incl. processed	Cherries	Grapefruit
Chicken	Dates	Honeydew
Cocoa, chocolate	Eggplant	Kale
Coffee	Eggs - chicken, duck	Kohlrabi
Corn	Figs	Lentils
Jam, jelly	Fish	Limes
Ice cream	Goat cheese	Mangos
Lard	Grapes	Mineral water
Lobster	Honey	Molasses
Mussels	Lemons	Mustard greens
Nuts	Lettuce	Nectarines
Oat bran	Maple Syrup	Onions
Oils - hydrogenated	Milk - cows, goat	Papayas
Peas - green, snow	Oatmeal	Peppers
Pork	Organic olive oil	Poppy seeds
Rye	Organic flaxseed oil	Raspberries
Soybeans, soy milk	Oranges	Sea salt
Sugar	Peaches	Sea vegetables
Veal	Pears	Soy sauce
	Pineapple	Sweet potatoes
	Plums	Tangerines
	Pumpkin	Watermelon
	Raisins	Yams
	Rice - wild, brown	
	Strawberries	
	Turkey	

Source: Colgan Institute, San Diego, CA.

'60s that confinement to bed can be fatal. In 10 weeks bed-rest patients lose 20 to 30% of their bone mass.[32]

Physicians, however, did not really appreciate (many still don't) the absolute need for daily weight-bearing exercise to grow bone, until America put men into space. Even though these young, super-healthy astronauts pedalled exercycles while in orbit, their bones melted away. Cycling can do wonders for the cardiovascular system, but, apart from the long bones of the legs, it does nothing to stress the skeleton. In their other activities, the weightlessness of space provided none of the pressure on the bone matrix essential to trigger the growth of new cells.[33]

Televison Causes Osteoporosis

Astronauts today do clever programs of daily resistance exercise in order to maintain their bones. But we Earthbound folk are not so smart. Mrs. Suburban Average gets no weight-bearing exercise. Instead, she watches television 5 - 8 hours a day. No wonder she's losing her bones.

With the information highway, virtual reality, and wall-size TV screens, soon we will be even more enticed to spend every waking hour interacting with a little beam of light - from the couch. By its creation of rampant couch potatoism, television is the biggest cause of osteoporosis in America. And it's totally man-made.

As usual, our health authorities have been tardy to recognize that excessive sitting in a chair causes disease. The US Academy of Sciences now agrees that weight-bearing exercise is essential to build and maintain bone strength.[20] But as recently as 1980, the **RDA handbook** made no mention of any form of exercise as being necessary for normal calcium metabolism.[34] And even today, the only therapies for osteoporosis approved by the FDA are calcium supplements and estrogen.

Many texts and osteoporosis advice booklets, such as the one I am holding now from the Washington State Dairy Council, recommend only walking or jogging. Or they vaguely refer to "exercise" as if any old activity will do.

We have already seen how cycling, running, walking and aerobics cannot do the job, because they mainly stress only the long bones of the legs. Other booklets I have recommend swimming, but it will not do either. As expert on osteoporosis, Dr. Robert Marcus of Stanford University School of Medicine says, swimming may be good for cardiovascular capacity, but it's a dud at protecting your bones, because it doesn't provide enough load.

You have to move some weight. But you don't need fancy exercise equipment. Your skeleton can't tell a gold-plated dumbell from a brick. Simply picking up a can of paint off the ground with both hands and extending it overhead stimulates all the major bones in your body.

Such stimulation certainly grows dense bone. At the Junior World Weightlifting Championships, researchers measured the bone strength of young weightlifters from 14 different countries, and compared them with healthy subjects who didn't lift weights. On average, the weightlifters bones were 46% more dense and an estimated 50% stronger.[35]

Recent studies also show that tennis players and baseball pitchers have stronger bones in their dominant playing arm.[36] Other important studies show that weight-bearing exercise has reversed osteoporosis,[37] whereas aerobic forms of exercise have no effect.[38]

In one study of older women, a year of aerobic exercise resulted in almost a 4% *loss* of bone mass. When weight-bearing exercises were added to the routine for the second and third years, the loss was reversed and the women gained a significant amount of bone.[39]

As the evidence piles up showing that regular weight-bearing exercise is essential for your bones, everyone is jumping on the weight-training bandwagon. The American College of Sports Medicine recently changed it's long time prescription of aerobic exercise to include exercise with weights. The Osteoporosis Society recommends exercise with weights. Even Ken Cooper, the aerobics king, has revised his programs to include weights. If you want to keep your bones, you should too. All you need to know about exercise is detailed in Chapter 25.

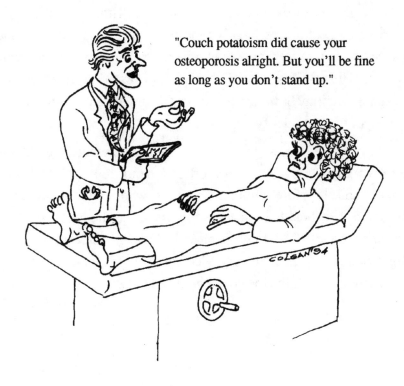

"Couch potatoism did cause your osteoporosis alright. But you'll be fine as long as you don't stand up."

Chapter 14

How Your Body Wears Out

The uninformed medical bureaucrats who have controlled 20th century health care largely ignored Nature. They viewed our reliance on the natural world as out-dated, and human science as all powerful. The result is blatantly before our eyes. Man-made chemicals and technology have turned our bodies and our environment into cesspools of rot and decay.

Fortunately, most of these men are now prematurely old, by their own hand. They are dying off and being replaced by better educated and therefore humbler scientists, who realize that human beings and their health are inextricably linked to the health of their environment and the nutrients it provides. We are entering the most enlightened era in human history. Medical science is finally accepting that Nature made all the locks and holds all the keys.

Miraculous Order

To take advantage of this new science, first you should understand how tightly your body is locked into Nature. Let's start at the beginning. In the middle of the morning on the second day of Creation, in the Archean era 400 million years ago, a miraculous combination of gases produced a few simple bacteria. My late mentor, Nobel Laureate physicist, Dick Feynman, convinced me it could not have been a random event. As a scientist, the best way I can describe it is this. A hand of intelligence reached into the chaos and the precise order of life was born.

At that time the atmosphere of the Earth was 98% carbon dioxide, plus a little methane and nitrogen. There was almost no oxygen.[1] The Archean bacteria began to "breathe" the carbon dioxide and produce oxygen as a waste product, as plants still do today. They multiplied across the face of the Earth. Over countless millennia, the carbon dioxide dwindled to its present fraction of 1%, and the atmosphere grew oxygen rich to its present 21%.[1]

This new abundance of oxygen made possible human life, but it poisoned the atmosphere for the bacteria that made it. They had to seek refuge in environments that are oxygen free. Today their progeny live on in the airless slime of river mud, and in the darkest recesses of the human gut.

These bacteria, that eons ago laid the groundwork for the creation of man, continue to support your life by their biological role in your intestines. Without them, along with some 40 other species of bacteria, with a combined weight about equal to the weight of your brain, you would degenerate and die.[2] This prime example of our dependence on ancient creatures underlines the precision of the design that binds together all life upon the Earth.

Natural Locks

You are locked into Nature and other organisms by a lot more than the oxygen they created and their function in your gut. The calcium of your bones was grown by the bodies of ancient marine life into their shells, that then became the soils from which the plants and animals we use as food now obtain their calcium. All the elements of your flesh have been precisely shaped and refined in this way in the bodies of thousands of creatures before you.

The sulfur in the proteins that comprise half the dry weight of your body, is taken from the soil by plants and washed into rivers by runoff. But it is never depleted. Why? Because of a minute phytoplankton that blooms in uncountable profusion over thousands of square miles of oceans. Every day **Emiliana huxleyii** produces millions of tons of **dimethyl sulfide**, which rises in evaporation of the surface water of the seas, and seeds the clouds with sulfur, which then precipitates on the land in rain. Without Emiliana most of mankind would sicken and die.[3]

We can track the course of nutrients through the ocean, through the air, through the soil, through the plants, through your body, and back to the ocean again. To the extent that this journey is unpolluted by toxic compounds, and undisturbed by the processing of foods, the nutrients themselves and the bodies that grow from them, remain healthy. To the extent that we deplete the nutrients, foul the air, pollute the water, degrade the soils, and contaminate the oceans, then your body is depleted and contaminated also, and pays the price in inevitable degeneration and disease.

Degeneration By Oxidation

To know how most human degeneration comes about, you have to understand a little about **oxidation**.

The rust that eats steel, the flaking of paint, the browning of cut apples, the rotting of meat, are all examples of oxidation. It is the most pervasive process of decay on Earth.

Oxidation is caused by **free radicals**, unstable atoms or molecules, usually of oxygen, that damage everything they touch. To dip into a smidgeon of physics, a stable atom always has its electrons in pairs to balance its nuclear forces. In contrast, the free radical has an unpaired electron in an outer orbit around its nucleus. This unstable configuration creates a powerful electromagnetic attraction that sucks an electron out of the nearest whole molecule of any material it touches. On losing an electron, that molecule then becomes a new free radical, which sucks an electron from the next whole molecule, and so on. This sequence continues many thousands of times, creating a free radical chain reaction of damage.

In 1957, Dr. Denman Harman at the University of Nebraska proposed that living flesh is also vulnerable to free radical attack.[4] So it has proved. We know now that most bodily damage involves oxidation. Ultra-violet light ages and decays your eyes and skin by oxidation. Air pollutants damage your lungs by oxidation. Many man-made drugs and chemicals tear your cells apart by oxidation. And, as we saw in earlier chapters, the main mechanism underlying cardiovascular disease and many cancers is - oxidation.

Don't despair. You can beat oxidation. The new nutrition science detailed in Chapter 20 can afford you lifelong protection.

Gravity Pulls You Down

The second big cause of aging and degeneration is gravity. Gravity is always trying to pull you out through the soles of your feet. You see double chins everywhere, but you never saw a double forehead. To combat gravity, you have to protect your skeleton and the muscles that hold it up.

The human body is designed to be almost continually active. Immobilize a joint for even a few hours and it starts to stiffen and decay. Disuse is deadly.

Under the usual medical treatment, a broken leg put in a cast loses most of its muscle, a third of its bone mass, and stiffens almost to immobility. Fortunately, the new medicine that is in concert with Nature, is now realizing how conventional medical technology causes more damage than it cures.

Confinement to bed, the conventional answer to many ills, is an example of the worst kind of treatment. In six months bed-rest you accelerate bone aging by a decade, losing 25-40% of your bone mass, much of it irreversible.[5]

The majority of skeletons and muscular systems of Mr. and Mrs. America degenerate prematurely, simply from our sedentary lifestyle. We get less and less active as we age, and lose the bulk of our muscle and bone. Dr. Walter Bortz of the Department of Medicine of the Palo Alto Medical Clinic in California, reviewed over 100 studies showing that many of the degenerative changes usually attributed to inevitable aging, are in fact caused by lack of exercise.[5]

Most Americans over 60 have insufficient muscle left to hold up their skeletons and insufficient bone mass to protect them against fractures. As we saw in Chapter 13, osteoporosis (weak bone disease) is now epidemic. More than 25 million Americans suffer this disease and it is growing silently in millions more. By our lack of understanding of Nature we are doing it all to ourselves. By age 65, one woman in every three suffers vertebral fractures. By age 80, one woman in three and one man in six suffers a hip fracture. They rarely recover mobility and a quarter of them die within six months.[6,7] Yet prevention is simple, costs nothing, and is available to everyone.

You can't avoid gravity, but you can combat it easily, even more easily than you can combat oxidation. Here's the clue. You sit like a slug, you grow like a slug. All you need to do is detailed in Chapter 25.

> If you have no time to exercise you'd better reserve a lot of time for disease.
> *Michael Colgan*
> *Nutrition Lectures, 1988.*

Chapter 15

Vitamins:
Nuts and Bolts
of Life

Vitamins are essential components of your body that it cannot make. You have to get them from your nutrition. As we have seen, our degraded food no longer contains sufficient vitamins for optimal health, and our needs for these nutrients are multiplied by the pollutants that pervade our food, water, and air. To meet these needs, the majority of Americans now take vitamin supplements, which are simply the vitamin components of our food, concentrated and made into pills or powders.

But many folk still see vitamins as some sort of drug, like caffeine or aspirin. They expect an immediate lift or an immediate reduction in pain or symptoms, and are disappointed when it usually doesn't happen. Let's get it straight. Vitamins are not stimulants, nor are they drugs for symptomatic relief. They are nutrients, and the business of nutrients is to *grow* a better body.

Growth Takes Time

Unlike drugs, whose fast and usually toxic action befits their intended use in crisis intervention, nutrients have few immediate effects that you can feel. Mostly they have to wait on Nature for deficient and defective cells to die off, and be replaced by new and better cells that grow from the improved nutrient mix.

You *can* use mega-doses of some nutrients to obtain quick, drug-like effects. Multi-gram amounts of niacin (vitamin B3) for instance, will reliably lower cholesterol levels, and some companies sell niacin supplements for this purpose. But, as with drugs, there is always a toxic downside. Mega-doses of niacin cause liver damage and cell destruction. Vitamin supplements are properly used for renewal of body tissues, never for their destruction.

Renewal is slow and steady. Your blood cells take three months for complete renewal. Many cells of your muscles and organs take six months. The matrix of your bones and teeth takes about a year.[1] That's what improved nutrition through supplementation is all about. You have to wait until the nutrients are built into your structure for their real benefits to show.

The neglected house plant provides a good analogy. If you start giving the plant a little TLC, seaweed fertilizer, and regular watering, the existing leaves and stems will perk up a bit. But to see the real benefit of your care, you have to wait as much as six months. You have to be patient until the old leaves and stems die off, and new ones sprout and flourish, with an improved cellular structure grown from the better nourishment.

Body Quality

Vitamins are the biochemical "nuts and bolts" that enable the proteins, carbohydrates, and fats of your tissues to function as a coordinated unit. Like the girders of a bridge, whose strength depends on the coordinated action of all the bolts acting together, so all the vitamins act in synergy with each other to provide optimal strength to your body. If even one vitamin is missing or deficient, it adversely affects the function of all the others.

Every year over 97% of your body is completely replaced, even the structure of the DNA of your genes, reconstructed entirely from the nutrients you eat. The quality of those nutrients determines the quality of your renewed cellular structure, the level at which it can function, and its resistance to disease. Any day that you are about to succumb to a fat-loaded hamburger or a nutritionless chocolate doughnut, think, "Do I really want this miserable excuse for food to become part of my flesh and my health tomorrow?"

If you seek the best of health and longevity, your answer should be a resounding, "No!" Instead you will eat nutrient-rich foods and will link and coordinate their action with vitamins. So that you know exactly what vitamins to take, this chapter answers these common questions about each:

- What does the vitamin do?

- What are the best food sources?

- Is the vitamin deficient in foods?

- What is the best supplement form of the vitamin and how much is safe and effective to take?

Vitamin A (Retinol)

Vitamin A is essential for normal vision, skin and mucous membranes, cell growth, reproduction and immunity to disease.[2] Retinol, named after the retina of your eye, is fat-soluble, meaning that it works in the lipids (fats) in your body. It also makes the visual purple of your eyes, essential for night vision.

Best food sources of vitamin A are liver and fish liver oils. Best sources of beta-carotene, which the body turns into vitamin A as needed, are carrots and green leafy vegetables.

Nationwide surveys find widespread vitamin A deficiency in the general public.[3]

Effective vitamin A supplements contain 5000-10,000 I.U. per day as retinol or palmitate. In some individuals vitamin A can build up in body fats to become toxic at or above an intake of 25,000 I.U. per day.[4] Large amounts of beta-carotene show little toxicity, apart from turning your skin as yellow as Tweety Bird.

Vitamin B1 (Thiamin)

Thiamin is a water-soluble vitamin, so it leaves the body daily and must be eaten daily. It is essential for energy metabolism, but, despite the claims of some supplement huxters, thiamin does not **create** more energy.

Best food sources of thiamin are whole grains. But losses of thiamin in the modern processing of grains into flour can be 100%.[5] Consequently, USDA surveys find that 45 of every 100 people are thiamin deficient.[6]

Effective supplements of thiamin range from 30-200 mg per day. Any supplement form is effective. Thiamin toxicity is zero even with supplements of 500 mg per day.[4] Capitalizing on this low toxicity, some so-called "energy" supplements contain gram amounts of thiamin and other B-vitamins. But even if you eat them till they come out your ears, they won't do a thing to fix the hitch in your giddy-up.

Vitamin B2 (Riboflavin)

Riboflavin is the second water-soluble B-vitamin. It helps the **mitochondria** (furnaces) of your cells to produce energy.

Best food sources are meats, poultry, fish and dairy foods. But processing food destroys up to 80% of the riboflavin content.[5]

Exercise dramatically increases your need for riboflavin. Even well-nourished athletes are sometimes deficient.[7]

Effective supplements of riboflavin range from 25-200 mg per day. Any form is effective. There are no reports of toxicity with this vitamin.[8]

Vitamin B3 (Niacin, Niacinamide)

Niacin is another water soluble B-vitamin. It works in the energy cycle and in tissue respiration.[9]

Best food sources of niacin are meats and fish. Niacin is not easily destroyed in food storage or processing.

Effective supplements of niacin range from 30-100 mg mostly as niacinamide. In the niacin form this vitamin causes a histamine release that makes your skin flush, burn and itch for up to three hours. Toxicity is low, but even 500 mg per day in the niacin form can cause liver inflammation.[4] It also causes you to look distinctly red-faced and irritable.

Vitamin B5 (Pantothenic Acid)

Pantothenic acid is a water-soluble B-vitamin that is essential for the body to make glycogen and fatty acids, your main fuels. It is also essential for making neurotransmitter chemicals that transfer information in your brain from one nerve to the next. Finally, it is essential for the body to make your steroid hormones, such as testosterone and estrogen.[9]

Pantothenic acid occurs widely in foods, with an average intake in America of 6 mg per day.[10] Obvious deficiency is uncommon. Some people appear to need a much higher intake for good health, especially if they are athletes or regular exercisers.

At the Colgan Institute we use 20-500 mg of the calcium pantothenate form or the pantothenic acid form with athletes. This vitamin is non-toxic even up to 10 grams per day.[11]

Vitamin B6 (Pyridoxine)

Pyridoxine is another water-soluble B-vitamin. It is essential for all stages of protein and amino acid metabolism, and in making hemoglobin, the oxygen carrying red pigment in your blood.

Best sources of pyridoxine are wheatgerm, chicken, fish and eggs. Despite its occurrence in all these foods, the Nationwide Food Consumption Survey showed that one-third of all American households are deficient in pyridoxine, even at the conservative RDA level of 2 mg per day.[12]

Requirements for this vitamin increase as energy expenditure and protein requirements increase, as they do in all regular exercisers. You cannot get toned and slim, nor put on a molecule of muscle, without sufficient pyridoxine.

Effective supplementation with pyridoxine requires 10-50 mg per day of pyridoxine hydrochloride, or the more expensive pyridoxal-5-phosphate. Despite the hype of some supplement makers, there is no advantage in the more expensive form, which is broken down into plain old pyridoxine in your gut. Intakes of over 100 mg per day for months can cause reversible nerve damage in some sensitive people.[13]

Vitamin B12 (Cyanocobalamin)

Probably the best known of the B-vitamins, cyanocobalamin is essential for every cell in your body, especially rapid turnover cells, including red blood cells and the lining of your intestinal tract.

The only sources of cobalamin are animal foods, so vegetarians are most commonly deficient. Average intake in America is 8 mcg per day for men and 5 mcg per day for women.[9] According to the **RDA handbook**, 3 mcg per day is sufficient to prevent a deficiency.

Injected mega-doses of cobalamin are used extensively to impart an inappropriate, but real, drug-like effect of increased energy. Even 10,000 times the RDA of cobalamin is non-toxic. No form of the vitamin has any advantage.

A very expensive and unstable form called dibencoside is sold with false claims that it is an energizer and an anabolic. To set the record straight, your body makes all the dibencoside it needs from vitamin B12 free of charge, so there is no need to pay for it.

Folate (Folic Acid, Folacin)

Folate, another B-vitamin, forms part of the transport coenzymes that control amino acid metabolism in your body. Deficiency of folate inhibits cell growth, especially growth of rapid turnover cells such as red blood cells.

Best sources of folate are fresh, dark-green leafy vegetables, beans and egg yolks. But even minimal food processing can destroy up to half the folate in your food.[9]

Government surveys show widespread folate deficiency in America, getting worse by the decade as our food becomes ever more processed and degraded.[9] The RDA for folate has been shamefully reduced by more than 50% as the available food folate has declined. The present RDA of 200 mcg per day has been shown in studies of sedentary people to put them in serious long-term deficit.[14]

Because use of large amounts of folate can mask the symptoms of pernicious anemia, the FDA restricts the maximum amount of folate per pill (dose) to 400 mcg per day (800 mcg during pregnancy). Even this higher figure may be insufficient for optimum health. At the Colgan Institute we have tracked healthy athletes for as long as four years, who have used 800 - 3400 mcg per day of folate with no side-effects. And a study of women given 10,000 mcg per day of folate for four months showed no ill-effects.[15]

Biotin

The last and most neglected of the B-vitamins, biotin forms part of enzymes essential for making of glycogen and fatty acids, your main fuels.

Best food sources of biotin are liver, sardines, egg yolks and soy flour.[9] The range of biotin in the American diet is 28-42 mcg per day.[16] RDA estimates of optimal intakes range from 100-300 mcg (**1980 RDA handbook**), to 30-100 mcg (**1989 RDA handbook**). Evidence favors the higher level, but the RDA Committee set the lower level in 1989 so that our degraded food supply wouldn't look so bad.

At the Colgan Institute we use 300-5000 mcg per day of biotin depending on the amount of exercise and the probable level of deficiency in the diet. No form is superior to any other, and 10,000 mcg per day shows no side-effects.[9]

Vitamin C (Ascorbate, Ascorbic Acid)

Like the B-vitamins, vitamin C is water-soluble, so it is quickly in and out of your body. Vitamin C is used in formation of collagen, the connective matrix of your flesh, and as an antioxidant to help protect you from oxidation.

Best sources of vitamin C are citrus fruits and leafy green vegetables, but it is easily destroyed by light, heat and chemicals. A fresh-cut lettuce for example, loses half its vitamin C in 48 hours, unless it is stored in a dark refrigerator.[5]

It takes only 30 mg per day of vitamin C to prevent scurvy, a disease of collagen breakdown. The average intake in America of 109 mg per day for males and 77 mg per day for females is well above this figure.[9]

But, as you will see in the antioxidant chapter, to be effective in preventing oxidation requires intakes of vitamin C in the multi-gram range. The greatest biochemist of the century, double Nobel Laureate Dr. Linus Pauling, first recommended multi-gram doses of vitamin C in the early '70s, and was rejected by the conservative scientific community of the time. Now in his 90s and still sharp as a tack, Pauling has long outlived his critics, and takes up to 18 grams of vitamin C daily in the multiple ascorbate forms.

At the Colgan Institute we use 2-12 grams of vitamin C per day. If taken as ascorbic acid, these amounts can cause stomach upsets in sensitive people. But taken as a mix of magnesium ascorbate, calcium ascorbate and the oil-soluble form ascorbyl palmitate, we have seen no detrimental side-effects. See the chapter on antioxidants for further information.

Vitamin D (Cholecalciferol)

Fat-soluble vitamin D is essential for bone growth and mineral balance in your body. Sunlight enables your skin to make vitamin D. Thirty minutes of summer sunshine on a body in a swimsuit produces many times more vitamin D than the RDA of 10 mcg. In the old IU units still appearing on labels, 40 IU = 1 mcg of vitamin D.

Vitamin D is added to milk and other foods so it is unlikely to be deficient in your diet. Supplements can become toxic if taken at five times or more of the RDA.[9]

Vitamin E

Fat-soluble vitamin E is mainly used by your body as an antioxidant.

Much of the vitamin E in foods is destroyed during processing. The amount left in American diets is about 10 mg alpha-TE (tocopherol equivalents).[9] This is the scientific measure which will replace the obsolete IU measure on labels. To help you translate, 1 mg alpha TE equals approximately 1 IU.

Because of the increased need for antioxidants in our polluted world, the Colgan Institute uses 400-2000 mg alpha-TE per day with athletes. Even 3000 mg-alpha TE, that is, 300 times the RDA, is non-toxic to most people.[17] Avoid the synthetic **dl** forms of vitamin E which contain unknown quantities of the inactive l-isomer. The best **d** form is natural source d-alpha tocopheryl succinate. Other natural tocopherols may also be biologically active.

Vitamin K (Phylloquinone)

Fat-soluble vitamin K is essential for formation of prothrombin, one of the compounds that enables your blood to clot. A vitamin K deficiency prevents the body from stopping bleeding in an injury.

Best sources of vitamin K are green leafy vegetables. The average American diet contains 300-500 mcg of vitamin K.[18] The RDA is only 80 mcg so you are unlikely to be deficient. Even mega-doses of the phylloquinone form of vitamin K have no reported toxicity.[9] But do not take supplements of the menadione form which can be very toxic.[19]

Choline

Choline is not a vitamin because your body can make it. Nevertheless most of your choline supply comes from your nutrient intake, so it is usually included in vitamin supplements. It's main function is as part of the brain neurotransmitter, acetylcholine. It also moves fats around the body.

Choline is widely available in foods, so deficiency is unlikely. Phosphatidyl choline is the best form. Even mega-doses of 20 grams are not toxic, but if taken in the choline chloride form will make you smell like rotting fish. Choline is often sold as a lipotropic, which people falsely translate as a fat-burner. Choline supplements have no effect at all on your level of bodyfat.

Inositol

Recent research shows that inositol is essential for normal calcium metabolism and insulin metabolism.[20,21] Inositol is also involved in fatty acid metabolism. Inositol is not a vitamin because your body can make it.

Along with choline, inositol is often falsely sold as a fat-burner.[22] It will not burn a molecule of your fat, but some folk find it useful in gram amounts for correcting mild insomnia. Even multi-gram doses do not produce toxic side-effects.[9]

Other Nutrients

Coenzyme Q10

Coenzyme Q10 (Ubiquinone) is essential for virtually all your energy production. It is also extensively used to maintain immunity,[22] heart function,[23] and as an antioxidant.[24]

Coenzyme Q occurs widely in foods and is converted in your body to coenzyme Q10. Your ability to make this conversion declines with age, so supplementation with the preformed Q10 is a sensible strategy for people past 35.

Despite volumes of evidence, the FDA has branded coenzyme Q10 supplements "unapproved food additives" in the US, although they are widely and successfully used in Europe and Japan to correct heart abnormalities.[23] At the Colgan Institute we use 10-60 mg of coenzyme Q10 per day. There is no toxicity at these levels of intake.

Bioflavonoids

This big family of compounds is under intense study as possible co-factors that increase the potency of anti-oxidants and for their actions against cancer and maintaining your cell membranes.[25]

Pyrolloquinolone Quinone (PQQ)

PQQ is a recently discovered nutrient involved in collagen metabolism.[26] Best food sources are fresh citrus fruits.

Para-amino-benzoic Acid (PABA)

We all know PABA because of its addition to sunscreens as a compound offering effective protection against ultra-violet B rays. In that context it does do something good. As a food supplement it has little to no support.

There are dozens of other similar compounds that are often added to supplements which have little or no evidence for their efficacy. So if you hear someone complain that I missed vitamin T or biopterin or other claptrap, smile to yourself that you know better. If it isn't noted in this chapter, there are no reliable scientific studies showing its value as a vitamin or vitamin co-factor, and you can safely ignore it.

> I've just left the FDA. It's the only thing to do when you wake up and find yourself there.
>
> *Name witheld*

Chapter 16

Minerals Are Your Framework

Ninety-six percent of your body is composed of five macro-elements, oxygen, hydrogen, nitrogen, carbon and sulfur. These are all abundant in the air you breathe and in your food. All proteins provide nitrogen for example, and the carbo bit of carbohydrates stands for the carbon they contain. You do not have to worry about getting sufficient macro-elements.

So what you usually see named as the essential minerals in food make up only a part of the remaining 4% of your flesh. Most of this tiny fraction, is composed of the macro-minerals, calcium, magnesium, phosphorous, potassium and chloride. Correct nutrition is vital to obtain sufficient macro-minerals because they are not abundant like the macro-elements.

Sixteen other minerals are also essential for optimal health, and the list increases every decade. These micro-minerals or trace elements occur in such tiny amounts in foods that correct nutrition becomes crucial in order to avoid deficiency. They are every bit as important as the macro-minerals. If even one micro-mineral is absent or deficient, then the function of all the other micro-minerals, macro-minerals and macro-elements is disturbed.

As with the vitamins, we will cover all the essential minerals under four headings:

- What does the mineral do?

- What are the best food sources?

- Is the American population deficient?

- What are the best forms to take and in what amount?

Calcium

A 145 lb body (70 kg) contains about 2.85 lbs (1.3 kg) of calcium, 99% of it in the bones and teeth. Most of the other 1% flows in and out of cells controlling conduction of impulses in nerves, contraction of muscles, and many other functions essential to continuing life. So whenever this vital 1% of calcium is not supplied by your nutrition, even for one day, your body cannibalizes it's own bones to make up the deficit.

A large glass of milk contains about 500 mg of calcium. Of that, 150 mg is absorbed. But milk is not a well tolerated food for adults and, because of our degraded food and dietary habits, average intake of calcium in America is only 743 mg per day.[1] That is way below the top RDA of 1200 mg.

Apart from people with a tendency to form calcium oxalate

kidney stones, calcium is non-toxic to at least 2500 mg per day.[1] At the Colgan Institute we use supplements of 400-1600 mg. Calcium citrate and calcium carbonate are good forms. Avoid bone meal, however, which is contaminated with lead.[2] Take all your mineral supplements together at night, because the mineral flux in the body that maintains bone growth is greatest during sleep.

Phosphorus

You have about 800 grams of phosphorus in your body, 700 grams of it in your bones.[1] The other 100 grams is essential for a multitude of purposes, from the energy cycle, to the formation of red blood cells.

Phosphorus is everywhere in foods and more is added during food processing. Best sources are meats, milk, fish and whole grains. Average daily intake in America is about 1500 mg for males and 1000 mg for females.[1] So deficiency is rare. Instead, because of food processing, Americans get a phosphorus overload.

The Colgan Institute does not use phosphorus supplements except as special ergogenic aids for athletes. Phosphorus is not toxic in multi-gram amounts, but does cause your body to lose calcium and also disrupts all other mineral metabolism. Our excess phosphorus additions to foods and as fertilizer are probably partly responsible for America's epidemic of osteoporosis.

Magnesium

Your body contains only 20-30 grams of magnesium, about an ounce. It forms part of over 300 vital enzymes as well as part of your bones. Magnesium is essential for burning of glycogen for fuel, muscle contraction, and transmission of the genetic code to form new proteins.

Best food sources of magnesium are whole grains and legumes. But over 80% of magnesium in grains is lost in removal of the germ and outer layers of grains to make refined white and so-called "enriched" flours. Don't eat them!

With the progressive degradation of our food, magnesium intakes have progressively declined in America. The average daily intake is now only 329 mg for males and 207 mg for females,[1] well below the RDA of 350 mg and 280 mg respectively.

Supplementation with magnesium as part of a complete mineral supplement is the only way to overcome this problem. The Colgan Institute uses 400-1200 mg per day of magnesium, preferably in the aspartate form. If your kidneys are healthy, there is no evidence of toxicity up to 6000 mg per day.[3]

Sodium

Sodium, potassium and chloride are your body's three main electrolytes. They perform multiple essential functions, without which your life would end in a heartbeat. Sodium is the main **cation** (positively charged electrolyte) outside cells.

So much sodium is added to our food that the average American eats about 5 grams per day, 10 times the recommended amount for good health.[1]

Never take salt pills and avoid all extra salt. Throw away your salt cellar or fill it with one of the alternative salts, especially one that is high in potassium. Excessive sodium raises blood pressure and has multiple other pathological effects. In our over-salted world, a low sodium diet is a basic principle of good health.

Chloride

Chloride is the main **anion** (negatively charged electrolyte) outside your cells. It works with sodium and potassium to regulate your fluid and electrolyte balance.

Along with our excessive sodium in salt added to our food, we also get excessive chloride, about 6 grams daily.[1] You need less than one gram daily. So don't take chloride supplements.

If you eat a low salt diet, then you get low sodium and low chloride intake, a wise dietary strategy.

Potassium

Potassium is the main **cation** (positively charged electrolyte) inside your cells. It interacts with sodium and chloride in conduction of nerve impulses and a host of other duties.

Good food sources of potassium are bananas and green leafy vegetables. Most fresh food, even fish, is high in potassium and low sodium. The average ratio of potassium to sodium is 7:1 in a mixed fresh food diet. Added sodium during processing reverses these ratios to 3.6 parts sodium to 1 part potassium, (see Chapter 2) leaving you swamped with sodium and deficient in potassium.

Average potassium intake in America has fallen to 2500 mg per day,[4] and much of that is lost again in people who use antibiotics or diuretics. The official recommended intake is 3500 mg per day. So Americans are considerably potassium deficient.

The Colgan Institute uses potassium supplements of 100-500 mg per day, preferably in the aspartate form. Potassium is not toxic up to about 5000 mg per day, but if taken without food can burn and upset your gut.

Iron

The main function of iron is in formation of hemoglobin, the oxygen-carrying red pigment in your blood.

Iron is widely available in foods, with **heme** iron from meats being the most bioavailable. Despite all the iron pills doled out in America, and the iron fortification of foods, many folk are deficient.[1] But do not take iron supplements except as part of a multi-mineral. Even 50 mg of iron by itself can be toxic. It is also hard for the body to get rid of, it is a potent source of bacterial growth, and it causes increased oxidation.

The Colgan Institute uses supplements of 10-25 mg of iron. The ferrous gluconate form is adequate and the iron picolinate form is very potent. But **never** take iron supplements except as part of a multi-mineral.

Zinc

Zinc forms part of many essential enzymes, that is, protein structures that catalyse (speed up) body functions, especially cell growth and immunity, testosterone production, sperm formation and sexuality.[5]

Bodily stores of zinc are small and have to be replaced constantly by zinc from your nutrition. Best sources are meats, eggs and seafoods. Studies of zinc intake in average diets show it is only 8.6 mg per day, well below the male RDA of 15 mg. Deficiency is rampant.

The Colgan Institute uses zinc supplements of 15-50 mg in the picolinate form. Toxicity of zinc is low, up to 500 mg per day.[3] But do not take zinc except as part of a multi-mineral supplement.

Excess zinc disrupts copper metabolism, which disrupts iron metabolism, which disrupts...... You get the picture. Excesses of single minerals are bad news.

Copper

Copper is essential for many enzymes including enzymes that help produce your hormones.

Best sources of copper are organ meats and seafoods. Average American diets provide 1.2 mg of copper per day for males and 0.9 mg for females.[6] The official recommended intake is 1.5-3.0 mg per day. So many folk are likely to be deficient, though copper deficiency is difficult to measure.

The Colgan Institute uses copper supplements of 0.5 - 3.0 mg in the sulfate form, to bring copper intakes up to the recommended level. Daily intakes of 10 mg show no toxicity.[3]

Manganese

You need manganese for proper formation of bone and for normal glucose metabolism. It also forms part of your internal antioxidant, superoxide dismutase.

Best food sources of manganese are whole grains and black tea. Average intake in America is 2.7 mg per day for men and 2.2 mg per day for women.[6] The amount of manganese required for optimum health is unknown. The **RDA handbook** recommends a provisional intake of 2 - 5 mg per day.[1]

The Colgan Institute uses supplements of manganese of 2 - 5 mg per day in the gluconate form. Manganese is one of the least toxic elements.

Chromium

Chromium is essential for glucose metabolism, insulin metabolism, fatty acid metabolism, and protein metabolism. It's a very important mineral.

Best sources of chromium are whole grains and shellfish. But up to 90% of chromium is lost in food processing.[7] Because of our food degradation, chromium is one of the most frequently deficient minerals in America. Average daily intake of chromium is only 25-33 mcg.[7] The **RDA handbook** recommends 50-200 mcg per day. So supplementation is essential for optimal health.

The Colgan Institute uses 200-800 mcg per day of chromium with athletes. The best form by far is chromium picolinate. Although it was developed only in the early '80s, chromium picolinate now has more than 40 research studies showing that it improves insulin metabolism, reduces bodyfat, increases lean muscle, and lowers cholesterol.[8] Chromium picolinate shows no toxicity even in amounts of 10-50 mg. Other chromiums, especially chromate, can be very toxic.

Selenium

Selenium forms part of key enzymes in the body for its work as an antioxidant.

Selenium is widespread in foods, but is deficient in the soils of ten states and the District of Columbia, so it is also deficient in the livestock and produce grown on those soils.[9] Average daily intake in America is about 108 mcg.[1] Because of our increased needs for antioxidants, this amount is likely to be insufficient.

The Colgan Institute uses 200-400 mcg per day of selenium

in the L-selenomethionine form. Selenium can be very toxic in excess of 800 mcg per day, especially in the sodium selenite form.

Iodine

Iodine is required to make your thyroid hormones, which in turn control all energy in your body.

Best sources of iodine are edible seaweed and seafoods. Even breathing sea air provides iodine. Deficiency is uncommon now because of iodized salt. But goitre and cretinism caused by iodine deficiency used to be common in Kentucky, Louisiana, Texas and South Carolina.[10] Average daily iodine intake in America is now 250 mcg for males and 170 mcg for females, well above the RDA of 150 mcg.

The Colgan Institue uses supplements of 50-200 mcg of iodine in the potassium iodide form with some athletes. Iodine is not very toxic up to 2000 mcg daily, but will exacerbate acne.

Boron

Boron was only recently shown to be essential for manufacture of some of your hormones.[11] Despite the hype of some supplement makers, however, boron is not anabolic, that is, does not cause muscle growth. Nor does it increase testosterone levels.

Boron occurs widely in foods in trace amounts, especially in soybeans, prunes, raisins, almonds and dates. Average daily intake in America is about 1.9 mg.[12]

Because of their greater hormone demands, the Colgan Institute supplements athletes with 3-6 mg of boron daily in mixed citrate and aspartate forms. Boron is a low-toxicity mineral, but intakes above 50 mg per day can interfere with phosphorus and riboflavin metabolism.[13]

Molybdenum

Molybdenum forms part of three essential enzymes.

Wholegrains and legumes are the best sources of molybdenum but amounts vary widely in these foods, depending on the molybdenum content of the soils in which they were grown. The amounts of molybdenum required for optimal health is unknown. Provisional RDA recommendation is 50-250 mcg per day.

The Colgan Institute uses 40-150 mcg per day in the sodium molybdate form, as part of a complete mineral supplement. Molybdenum is not toxic up to 9 mg per day. Above that it causes a gout-like condition.[14]

Other Minerals

Studies indicate that **silica** (more properly silicon) is essential for normal bone growth. **Cobalt** forms an essential part of vitamin B_{12}. **Nickel** and **arsenic** are essential for normal growth in animals. And there is mounting evidence that **tin**, **germanium**, and **vanadium** may be required in minute amounts.[11]

The operative words for these last three are minute amounts. Supplements of vanadium and germanium now being touted in the market-place are just modern variants of snake oil. When you paid your buck to the carpetbagger on the boardwalk, you knew it was really a fee to see him perform. You threw away the musty bottle of goop, or gave it to your mother-in-law. But today snake oil comes in shiny packages with all the bells and whistles of Madison Avenue pseudoscience. Read this book well to avoid the scams. And, if still in doubt, look up the medical references that support what I say. That way you'll save both your money and your health.

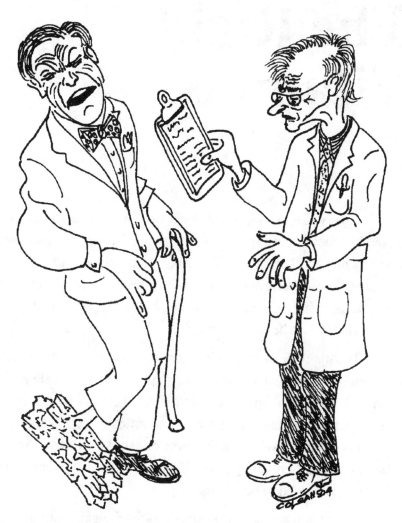

"First you gave me calcium, then magnesium, then silica - and now look what's happened!"

Chapter 17

The Right Vitamins

Every drug store, health food store and supermarket today presents a bewildering array of vitamins, minerals, and other supplements, all claiming to be the best. How do you know which ones are true-to-label, potent, made of the best forms of the nutrients and right for you? This chapter tells you how to separate the few that are excellent from the masses of ugly.

The majority of multi-vitamins are woefully inadequate. In a recent study at Yale New Haven Hospital, researchers evaluated all common brands of vitamins bought off the shelf at a wide range of stores. Many were made with the wrong ratios of nutrients to each other, or contained too little of the more expensive nutrients, or were missing some nutrients altogether. Of the 257 vitamin products tested, only 49 were judged to be adequate.[1]

We have done similar analyses at the Colgan Institute since 1982. We buy samples of the products like you do - off the store shelf. No manufacturers pay us to test their products, and we receive no federal grants or other monies for this work. It is part of our nutrition education function.

We maintain a hotline used by many thousands of people, researchers, agencies, on which we will tell you which brands of supplements we have tested and which ones we recommend. The office number is (619)632-7722.

From us you will get the truth, not the clever hyperbole you see on television and in the newspapers. Look at Centrum for example, the most advertised vitamin on TV. Capitalizing on the mass of new evidence that antioxidants prevent disease, the ads say, "Contains the complete antioxidant group." True, but in what amounts. When you read the small print on the label it says, vitamin C, 60 mg. Yet the studies showing disease prevention effects of vitamin C almost all involve gram amounts, 20-100 times the amount in Centrum.

For vitamin E the Centrum label says 30 IU. Yet the studies show that disease prevention effects of vitamin E require over 100 IU. Beta-carotene is the same story. Centrum contains 1000 IU, whereas studies finding preventive effects of beta-carotene involve 20-50 times this amount.

I am not singling out Centrum. It's just a brand everyone knows. As an all round multi-vitamin Centrum is better than most. I am simply telling you the truth.

Price of Nutrients

Effective potency is only the first problem. Different nutrients vary widely in price. Iron sulfate for example, costs only pennies, whereas pure biotin costs around $6000 per pound, wholesale. You can guess how that influences formulations.

Different forms of the *same* nutrient can also cover a 20-fold range in price. A pill reading, "Vitamin E as mixed tocopherol complex, 400 IU", can contain anything from a cheap blend of 50% tocopherols and 50% vegetable oil, to a very expensive blend of 95% tocopherols and 5% vegetable oil. The only guide you have as a consumer is the retail price.

But price is not infallible. Some companies, with lots of hype, sell dibencoside for example, a very expensive form of vitamin B_{12}. But dibencoside is broken down by digestion into plain old vitamin B_{12}, so it is no better than the regular form.

Pyridoxal-5-phosphate, (P-5-P), an expensive form of vitamin B_6, is the same. Marketers of supplements cite studies on the benefits of *injected* P-5-P. But in pill form it is broken down to plain old vitamin B_6 by your digestion. So inexpensive pyridoxine hydrochloride is just as good.

The only way you can know the truth about these and many other forms of nutrients is to ask independent experts, such as the Colgan Institute, who have spent a lifetime in nutrition research. Unlike corporate, government, and university scientists, most of whom are biased by fear of losing profits, status, or research grants, we will tell you the truth.

No Natural Vitamins

Many companies falsely label their supplements "natural" because the word sells. Let's get it straight. Vitamin pill ingredients today are about as natural as a polyester suit. Manufacturers dodge around this issue with phrases like "natural grown", "natural source", "food grown", but the truth is, most pill ingredients are synthetic. That is, they are natural materials (what else is there) treated with various chemical procedures, so that their resemblance to the natural material is remote.

Most vitamin C for example, is made from corn. First the corn is chemically converted to sugar (d-ribose). Then the sugar is chemically converted to pure, ascorbic acid. There is not a molecule of corn left in it. It is the chemical processing that makes it synthetic, not the raw materials it came from.

What about "natural rose hip" or "acerola" vitamin C. The best rose hip and acerola powders contain only a few milligrams of vitamin C per gram. A 1000 mg pill of natural rose hip vitamin C would be about the size of a baseball. All these so-called "natural" pills are predominantly synthetic ascorbic acid, with a pinch of the natural powder thrown in for marketing.

Then there are those companies who claim that their pills are made of superior vitamins. Let's get this one straight too. Almost all the vitamin raw materials in America come from a few large companies. Hoffman La Roche makes most of the vitamin C and many of the B-vitamins. Henkel makes most of the vitamin E. Almost all pill manufacturers buy their bulk powders from the same sources that are available to everyone.

Elemental Minerals

Most consumers don't know that chemical forms of minerals are not elemental forms. A 1200 mg pill of calcium gluconate for example, is only 9% elemental.[2] That is, it contains only 108 mg of calcium. To get the RDA for calcium, you would have to swallow eleven of these pills every day.

The same goes for every mineral. Calcium citrate is only 21% calcium. Chromium picolinate is only 12½% chromium.

Magnesium aspartate is only 11% magnesium. Some forms contain only 1-2 % of the mineral element. Manufacturers are supposed to state the elemental amounts on the label, but many do not.

Chemical Forms

By law, supplement pills only have to be true to label chemically. That is, if the bottle says the pill contains say 300 mg of magnesium, that is all it has to do. But many chemical forms of nutrients are hardly bioavailable at all. They pass right through your intestines without ever being absorbed.

Magnesium supplied as magnesium oxide for example, is only one-tenth as bioavailable as magnesium aspartate. But the aspartate form is more expensive than the oxide and takes up more room in the pill. Manufacturers can save money by using the oxide. They can also fit more magnesium into a given size pill by using the oxide, and therefore can put a bigger number for magnesium on the label. Consumers go for big numbers.

Some manufacturers fudge bioavailability by claiming particular absorption rates, such as 60%, for their multi-nutrient supplements. All such claims are false, because different nutrients and different forms of the same nutrient are all absorbed at different rates. An average absorption rate is advertising nonsense.

Of a 100 mcg vitamin B_{12} tablet for example, only about 3% is absorbed, whereas calcium acetate is 32% absorbed.[2] To say the average absorption rate is 17½% for the two combined, tells you nothing about either.

One reason I wrote this book was to help steer the public through the maze of supplement gobbledegook. You can also call the Colgan Institute at (619)632-7722. If you want the best of health, use both sources well.

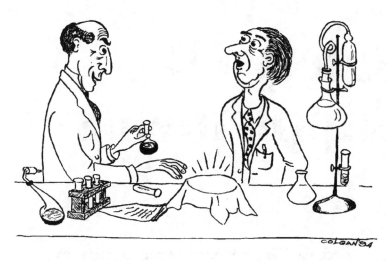

"I've invented a complete mutli-vitamin pill you only have to take once a month."

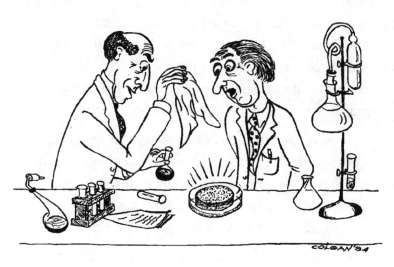

"I just have to cut down the size a bit."

Chapter 18

Safety Of Supplements

Since the Colgan Institute opened in 1974, we have used nutrient supplements with over 32,000 people. Many of these people have been taking them regularly for the whole 20 years of our existence. During that time we have had 231 cases of reported nutrient toxicity. We analyze each case of possible toxicity with great care. We have found that 189 cases were not caused by the nutrients, but by traumas, foods eaten at the time, coincidental infections, illnesses, or emotional stress. In most cases symptoms disappeared over time despite continued supplement use.

In 40 of the remaining cases symptoms disappeared on cessation or reduction of the supplements. Twenty-nine of them were real reactions to the nutrients involving skin rashes, gastrointestinal upsets, headaches, nausea or fatigue. None was serious. Only two cases had to cease taking supplements permanently.

Two out of 32,000 over 20 years is an enviable record. If our experience reflects the safety of sensibly used supplements, then they are a lot less toxic than the American food supply. The Centers for Disease Control for example, report that *half* of all raw chicken and eggs sold in America are contaminated with salmonella or campylobacter. These toxic bacteria *kill* 2000 Americans every year and poison six million of us.[1] Supplements are a lot safer than that.

Prescription Drugs Are The Poisons

Uninformed national media love to engage in vitamin bashing, and any case of supposed toxicity is eagerly seized on. Over the years vitamin A has been called a poison by the FDA, vitamin C has been accused of destroying vitamin B12, and of causing rebound scurvy when you stop taking it, and vitamin B6 has been denounced as a cause of nerve damage.

The Colgan Institute investigated each of these claims. The gist of these investigations is covered in my book, **Optimum Sports Nutrition.**[2] The vitamin C claims of toxicity are blatantly false. The vitamin A and vitamin B6 claims of toxicity do not apply to any reasonable dose. Our research only serves to confirm what Ernest Hemingway said long ago, if you rely on newspapers, you develop a newspaper intelligence.

Remember, anything can be toxic, even water, if you take enough of it. In Chapters 15 and 16, I specify the dosages we use of every vitamin and mineral, and the massive doses that you have to take, to no good purpose, in order to cause toxicity. The amounts we use are well supported by research, and have not caused any toxicity problems in many thousands of people for the last 20 years.

But do not take my word for it. The strongest evidence for the safety of nutrient supplements is found in the annual reports of the Poison Control Centers.[3] For the years 1985-1990, poison emergencies with medical drugs killed 2251 people. Simple anal-gesics, such as aspirin killed 640 people.

I say emergencies because the number of deaths caused each year by "normal" use of medical drugs is enormous. In hearings before Rep. Elton Gallegly on 18 February 1994, Mitchell Zeller of the FDA coolly announced that the number of deaths in America from "normal" use of prescription drugs is an estimated 150,000 per year. That is an obscene 900,000 deaths between 1985 and 1990. Publicly, the FDA keeps very quiet about these figures, because they approved the prescription drug use in the first place.

In the same period, the nutrient supplements now used by more than 100 million Americans every day, killed *one* person - by overdose of niacin. Used in any sensible amounts, vitamins and minerals are about as toxic as apple pie.

> The only differences between drugs and poisons are dosage and intent.

Chapter 19

Nutrition Is The New Medicine

The last five years have seen the most profound change in medical attitudes towards nutrition. On 19 August 1992, for the first time in its history, the ultra-conservative **Journal of the American Medical Association** recommended vitamin supplements as a way to prevent atherosclerosis and heart disease.[1]

Then in May 1993, the highly respected **New England Journal of Medicine** published two large population studies, involving 130,000 health workers showing that high doses of vitamin E significantly reduce risks of heart attacks and strokes in both men and women.[2,3] The researchers showed that it was next to impossible to get sufficient vitamin E from our food and, with the agreement of the journal's conservative editors, made a clear recommendation for vitamin E supplementation.

In a special editorial by Dr. Daniel Steinberg of the University of California, San Diego, the **New England Journal of Medicine** itself boosted the recommendation. Steinberg reviewed the lack of toxicity of vitamin E and posed the rhetorical question. "Should we recommend that our patients take antioxidant supplements?" His reply, "Why not?", although hedged with caveats, was clearly positive.

Then the scholarly journal, **Nutrition Reviews**, the bible of nutrition science used by researchers themselves, and the pinnacle of scientific respectability, joined the fray. It showed unequivocally that it is impossible to get sufficient vitamins from our degraded food supply, and criticized the FDA for failing to permit companies to tell the public how vitamins prevent cancer.[4]

The **New England Journal of Medicine** concurred with a massive study of 89,000 female nurses followed for 8 years. The research showed that those nurses whose intakes of vitamin A were 30% greater than the RDA, or higher, had significantly less risk of breast cancer.[5]

Not to be left out of the female cancer debate, the **Journal of the American Medical Association** published a study by Dr. Charles Butterworth of the University of Alabama School of Medicine. The study showed clearly that women with deficient intakes of the B-vitamin folate (as we saw in Chapter 15, a very common deficiency in America), had no resistance to the papilloma virus that causes cervical cancer. Folate deficiency was shown to be a worse risk for cervical cancer than smoking.[6]

These are a tiny sample of the hundreds of recent reports in mainstream medical journals showing that decent nutrition that includes vitamin and mineral supplements is a major force in preventing a wide range of degenerative diseases, including most cancers, cardiovascular diseases, adult-onset diabetes, and many liver, kidney, skin, eye and other organ disorders. But don't just listen to me. Read the medical references that I cite. Even the small sample listed in this book are enough to convince you to take care of your nutrition lifelong.

Negative Findings

Of course there are some negative reports about vitamins. And they get disproportionate media coverage because media administrators love vitamin bashing. The powerful pharmaceutical advertisers don't look kindly on media that applaud non-patentable vitamins to prevent illness, because their bottom lines depend on an ever increasing number of people becoming dependent on patented prescription drugs.

As I am writing this chapter, national media are being cleverly manipulated to misinterpret a new study appearing today (14 April 1994) in the **New England Journal of Medicine**. This study, sponsored by the US National Cancer Institute, examined the effects of beta-carotene and vitamin E on 29,000 smokers aged 50 and above. After 5-8 years, researchers reported they could find no evidence of a reduction in the risk of lung cancer.[7]

The widely quoted comments about this study by allegedly responsible people, such as Dr. Gilbert Omenn, Dean of Public Health of the University of Washington in Seattle, are particularly disturbing. I hope Dr. Omenn was misquoted when he claimed that the study applies to healthy people, "because smokers get the same diseases as the rest of us".[8]

The study has no application whatsoever to healthy folk. Study subjects were all long-term, heavy smokers, all over age 50.

At the start of the study, the men averaged 57.2 years of age, smoked an average of 20.4 cigarettes a day, and had smoked for an average of 35.9 years.[7] As we saw in Chapter 12, most cancers grow silently for many years before emerging as symptoms or bodily changes that are detectable. The disease processes caused by smoking were already well advanced in these men before the study began. To then give them a modicum of vitamins and expect a cure is non-sensical. It shows about the same intelligence as taking aspirin to cure a rotting tooth.

The study has little application even to smokers. The media reports fail to cite the amounts of vitamins used. Amounts were negligible. The 50 mg of synthetic dl-alpha tocopherol acetate per day in the study, (50 IU)[9] is a miniscule amount, and the poor synthetic form to boot. To put it in perspective, a bowl of wheatgerm cereal contains about 20 IU of vitamin E.[10] A recent review of all the major studies in the conservative **Journal of the American Dietetic Association**, recommended 200-800 IU of vitamin E per day for health protection. And that is for ***non-smokers***.[11]

Similarly, the 20 mg of beta-carotene (33,320 IU)[9] per day in the study, affords very little protection against the massive disease processes already at work in subjects who have smoked heavily for many years. Twenty milligrams of beta-carotene is only the amount in two large carrots.

Smoking is a deadly practice. Remember, cigarette packets carry the Surgeon General's warning: "Smoking Causes Lung Cancer . . .". Not ***might*** or ***can*** cause lung cancer but does - period! To suggest you can stop this disease process with a couple of carrots a day is ludicrous.

After reviewing all the relevant studies, the Colgan Institute uses 25,000 - 50,000 IU of beta-carotene per day (15-30 mg) for normal health maintenance in healthy people. Smokers would need a lot more than that to effectively combat their condition.

If ever a study was designed to fail, this was it. The researchers should be ashamed of themselves. But it's no surprise that our $43 million dollars of tax money was spent on work of such outstanding brilliance and perspicacity. As we saw in Chapter 12, the National Cancer Institute has made many similar "mistakes" in the past. This 2-billion-a-year mega-institution does not want its power and income eroded by cancer prevention strategies that the public can use by themselves.

Don't take my word for it. If you want the nitty-gritty on the activities of the National Cancer Institute, get **The Politics of Cancer** by Samuel Epstein, Professor of Medicine at the University of Illinois. Dr. Epstein shows clearly how ineffectual our cancer health authorities are today.[12] The Colgan Institute receives numerous press releases and reports from the National Cancer Institute. We read them all carefully, but have long since ceased believing in most of what they say.

Authorities Approve Vitamins

For the truth about vitamins, look to experts whose status and salary does not depend on continuing disease. The evidence has now convinced thousands of the leading scientists in America. And, despite the risks to their university careers and federal research grants, those with enough guts and integrity are saying so in the public media.

Let's look at a few of their comments. Jerome Cohen MD, Professor of Internal Medicine at St Louis University School of Medicine used to be against vitamin supplements. Now he will tell you he takes 400 IU of vitamin E daily to help protect his heart.[13]

Dr. Simin Meydani of the Human Nutrition Research Center on Aging at Tufts University, Boston: "We used to think of vitamins strictly in terms of what you needed to prevent short-term deficiencies. Now we are starting to think about what is the optimal level of vitamins for lifelong health and to prevent age-associated diseases."[14]

To demonstrate the effects of vitamin C, Dr. Gladys Block, formerly of the National Cancer Institute, now at the University of California, Berkeley, reviewed the 15 top studies on vitamin C and cancer rates. People in the top 25% regarding vitamin C intake, had only one-half to one-third the rate of cancers of the esophagus and stomach of those in the bottom 25%.[15]

Dr. Daniel Menzel of the University of California at Irvine: "Priming children with antioxidants could protect them against lung disease as adults...".[16]

Eminent researcher Dr. Walter Willett of Harvard: "Until quite recently, it was taught that everyone in this country gets enough vitamins through their diet and that taking supplements just creates expensive urine. I think we now have proof that this isn't true. I think the scientific community has realized this is a very important area for research."[13,16]

My computer files contain masses of such public acclamation from eminent scientists, but space restricts how many I can include here. Those I have quoted are representative, though they only scratch the surface of the huge vitamin revolution now happening in America. As a 20-year researcher in the field myself, it gladdens my heart to see that this vital health information is finally getting out to the public.

Sixty percent of all Washington State dieticians now take multi-vitamins for example.[17] And a new poll shows that 78% of Americans now believe that taking supplements will help maintain their health.[18] The prestigious **Kellogg Report** estimates that dissemination of new nutrition information will save $20.5 billion in health care costs.[18]

So strong is the evidence and the public approval of supplements, that some State governments are considering putting them under insurance coverage in the new legislation required to introduce the Clinton health care plan. Vermont has already jumped the gun with a bill proposing tax deductions for vitamin supplements.[19]

I've saved the best for last in this chapter. For years I have watched the evidence in favor of vitamins grow and grow. For years I have recorded the guarded but gradually changing public statements of the top researchers at the premier government nutrition research organization, the USDA Human Nutrition Research Center. On 4 March 1994 their Director of Antioxidant Research, Dr. Jeffrey Blumberg, as conservative and careful a scientist as I've ever known, finally said it straight. Talking about supplements of vitamins C and E and beta-carotene, he said, *"We have the confidence that these things really do work."*[20] The following chapters get down to the details.

Our current health-care crisis is the culmination of public despair at the inability of our medical priesthood and its high technology religion to perform miracles with bodies that are already in death's boat and halfway across the Styx.

Michael Colgan
Medical Lectures, 1994.

Chapter 20

Antioxidants Against Disease

The evidence is now irrefutable that the right use of the right antioxidants can prevent and even reverse many forms of cancer, heart disease, atherosclerosis, adult-onset diabetes, and a host of other diseases whose primary cause is excess oxidation, including cataracts, lung disorders, liver disorders and degenerative diseases of the brain.

These are big claims, so I better provide strong evidence to support them. I can only cover a small fraction of the studies here, so will focus on a selection of the latest and best.

The major antioxidants and their co-factors are listed in Table 8 in the forms and amounts used by the Colgan Institute and other laboratories in studies that have successfully inhibited a wide variety of diseases, and have also improved the vitality and performance of folk already in excellent health.

Table 8: Antioxidants used in medical studies and studies with athletes.

Nutrient	Daily Amount
N-acetyl cysteine*	50-350 mg
L-glutathione	100-200 mg
Vitamin A (palmitate)	5000-10,000 IU
Beta carotene**	10,000-25,000 IU
Vitamin C as:	
ascorbic acid	2000-10,000 mg
calcium ascorbate	500 - 1000 mg
magnesium ascorbate	500-1000 mg
ascorbyl palmitate	250-500 mg
Vitamin E as:	
tocopherol complex	200-800 IU
d-alpha tocopheryl succinate	400-1200 IU
Zinc (picolinate)[§]	10-60 mg
Selenium[‡] as:	
selenomethionine	200-400 mcg
sodium selenite	100-200 mcg
Co-Enzyme Q10	30-60 mg

* N-acetyl cysteine should be used only with at least three times its amount of vitamin C, so as to avoid the possibility of it precipitating in the kidneys as cystine, and possibly causing kidney stones in sensitive individuals.

** Beta-carotene is a safe source of vitamin A at the levels given. Vitamin A may become toxic beyond 25,000 IU per day.

§ Zinc acts as an antioxidant co-factor.

‡ Selenium can become very toxic over 800 micrograms per day, especially in the inorganic form of sodium selenite.

Source: Colgan Institute, San Diego, CA.

I have to note that the FDA may soon ban **coenzyme Q10** from the American market, yet another example of their inestimable wisdom. This innocuous nutrient is used successfully throughout the rest of the civilized world to treat various oxidation conditions, and is prescribed in Japan for heart disease. Anyone who did not believe in the unwavering integrity of our health authorities, might think that the FDA action is motivated by pharmaceutical conglomerates who are working to gain approval for prescription only coenzyme Q10 in the US. Heaven forbid!

Another FDA threatened nutrient on the list, **l-glutathione** ,is the only endogenous antioxidant you can use as an oral supplement. Your body makes l-glutathione from the non-essential amino acids l-cysteine, glutamic acid, and l-glycine. But evidence indicates that the body does not make sufficient l-glutathione to inhibit particular types of oxidation, especially as we age.[1] **N-acetyl cysteine** provides a good oral base for l-glutathione, which is why we also include it in the antioxidant mix.

The other two major endogenous antioxidants, superoxide dismutase, and catalase, are also sold as oral antioxidant supplements but only by the unscrupulous. These are bogus products. As I show in my book **Optimum Sports Nutrition**, both are destroyed by digestion and the first pass through your liver.

The ranges of antioxidants shown in Table 8 are averages extracted from more than 500 successful studies. No one knows the amounts of antioxidants required for optimal health, so we have to rely on successful studies, both with diseases and with healthy folk such as athletes, to give us guidelines to antioxidant use that is effective and without toxicity.

Before we go any further, long-term use of antioxidant

supplements is still an experiment. The safety of amounts shown here has not been confirmed by long-term trials in humans. Also, these amounts are used with patients and with athletes, whose bodies are under far more stress than the bodies of average folk, and therefore require increased amounts of nutrients. We would not use any more than the lower figures with recreational athletes, and Table 8 is not a recommendation to you to use even those amounts.

If you review the medical references given and decide to use antioxidants, then it is at your own choice and risk. All I can tell you is that I, my family and friends, and thousands of clients of the Colgan Institute worldwide, have used antioxidant supplements for the last 20 years, and we have used them in our research, with no evidence of toxicity and great evidence of benefit.

Antioxidants Prevent Cancer

The latest study in the **Journal of the American Medical Association** shows unequivocally that the incidence of cancer is rapidly increasing in America. Head researcher on the study, Dr. Devra Davis and her colleagues, conclude that the cancer increase probably results from our increasing exposure to carcinogens in the environment, including pesticides, herbicides, chemical solvents, tobacco, and industrial and auto emissions.[2] Just what I've been saying throughout this book. Let's see how antioxidants and lifestyle changes can protect you.

The worst cancer risk is smoking, including second-hand smoke. Like most pollutants, it damages you mainly by oxidation. In combination with other air pollutants, smoking is now linked to 33% of all cancers.[3] But I hope that you don't smoke, and you avoid anyone who does.

The next big cancer risk is overweight. In 1959 the American Cancer Society began a massive study of over a million Americans in 25 states. At the end of the study in 1980, results showed that men and women who are 40% or more overweight have higher rates of a wide variety of cancers.[4] The evidence suggests that many of these cancers occur because of lipid oxidation, that is, excess fat molecules in your body go rancid and initiate cell damage that progresses into cancer.

To the average person in my lectures, pesticides seem a bigger cancer threat than overweight. In fact cancer risk from too much bodyfat is many times that of all the pesticides put together. Approximately 24% of all cancers are linked to obesity.[5] But, don't despair. Chapter 24 shows you how to conquer the flab once and for all.

Vitamin A Prevents Cancer

Let's highlight the evidence that particular antioxidants can save you from cancer. In an authoritative review of all major studies on vitamin A, Dr. Thomas Kummet and Dr. Frank Meyskins of the University of Arizona conclude, *"a protective effect of vitamin A has been found for almost all sites of cancer"*. [6]

The most recent large, controlled study followed 89,000 female nurses for eight years. Those with intakes of vitamin A above 6630 IU per day had significantly lower incidence of cancer. The RDA for vitamin A is only 5000 IU per day, and the average American intake is only about 3900 IU. If you are among the average - Good Luck!

Beta-Carotene Prevents Cancer

Beta-carotene (the precursor of vitamin A), is the most prevalent source of vitamin A in our food. Many of the studies are therefore measuring mostly beta-carotene, but they report it as units of vitamin A activity. Lucky for us, because recent work shows that beta-carotene has a stronger effect against cancer than vitamin A itself.[7,8] This is a great discovery because high intakes of vitamin A (above 10,000 IU per day) can be toxic in sensitive individuals, whereas beta-carotene rarely shows any toxicity.

In a masive test of beta-carotene, Japan studied 250,000 people as part of the census. The analysis showed that people with diets low in beta-carotene had increased risks of lung cancer, stomach cancer, colon cancer, prostate cancer, and cervical cancer.[9]

Both the National Cancer Institute and the American Cancer Society now accept that beta-carotene protects you against cancer. But the average beta-carotene intake in American adults is only about one-third of the amount recommended by the National Cancer Institute to prevent cancer.[10] If your intake is average, and you cannot bring yourself to change, then a quick deposit on a cemetery plot may be your best course of action.

Vitamin C Prevents Cancer

Does vitamin C also prevent cancer? You bet! Cancer expert Dr. Bruce Ames at the University of California, Berkeley, reviewed a mass of animal studies showing protective effects of vitamin C against a wide variety of cancers.[11] And Dr. E. Bjelke at the University of Minnesota, showed that men with high intakes of vitamin C had much lower incidence of stomach cancer, colon cancer, and rectal cancer.[12]

The amount of vitamin C necessary to prevent cancer is much higher than can be provided by the American food supply. The latest **RDA handbook** shows that average intake of vitamin C in America is 109 mg/day for men and 77 mg for women.[13] Yet the amount of vitamin C used in studies that successfully inhibit formation of carcinogens is in the ***multi-gram*** range.[14]

Vitamin E Prevents Cancer

Vitamin E has similar protective effects. Dr. Paul Knekt and colleagues studied 21,000 men for 10 years. Those with high intakes and high blood levels of vitamin E showed a 30% lower risk of all types of cancer.[15]

Another well controlled study followed 15,000 women for eight years, who all initially showed no evidence of cancer. Those women in the group with low blood levels of vitamin E, developed 160% more cancers during the follow-up.[16]

As with vitamin C, the amounts of vitamin E required to prevent cancer are much larger than can be provided by our food, even if you follow the Eating Right Pyramid to the letter. Average vitamin E intake in America is only 7-11 IU per day.[13] A recent study in the conservative **Journal of the American Dietetic Association** recommended 200-800 IU of vitamin E per day to obtain protective effects.[17]

Some uninformed media have suggested that 800 IU or more of vitamin E is toxic, raises blood pressure, and commits all manner of mischief in the human system. ***Don't believe them.*** Experts on vitamin E, Drs. Lawrence Machlin and Adrienne Bendich, reviewed all the human studies on vitamin E use, and concluded that even 3200 IU daily for six months showed negligible toxic effects on subjects in normal health. [18]

Selenium Prevents Cancer

Cancer expert Dr. Bruce Ames, Professor of Biochemistry at UC Berkeley in San Francisco, reviews extensive animal studies showing that selenium inhibits development of deliberately induced cancers of the breast, liver, skin and colon. [19]

It works in men too. In a massive study, Dr. Paul Knekt and colleagues in Finland took and froze serum samples from 21,172 men. Over the next decade, 143 developed lung cancer. When the stored serum samples were analyzed and compared with a control group, the cancer victims showed much lower selenium levels than controls. [20]

Selenium deficiency affects more than your lungs. Dr. V. Reinhold and colleagues in the Department of Dermatology at the University of Bonn have found similar effects with the deadly skin cancer melanoma. They examined the serum of melanoma patients and compared it with controls. The cancer patients showed significantly lower levels of selenium, even in early stages of the disease.

These findings indicate that the deficient selenium nutrition *preceded* the melanoma. Selenium is known to protect skin from ultra-violet damage, which, as we have discussed, occurs by oxidation. So it is likely that the selenium deficit was a primary cause of the cancer. [21]

This study is especially important, because our careless use of **chlorofluorocarbons** has destroyed part of the ozone layer protecting the Earth from ultra-violet light. The Environmental Protection Agency predicts over one million additional cases of skincancer in America before the end of the century, caused directly by the depletion of ozone. No one can protect you except yourself. It seems only common sense to ensure an adequate intake of selenium.

How much is adequate? A difficult question because selenium in the sodium selenite form can be toxic, even a daily intake of only one milligram. The National Academy of Sciences suggests 50-200 micrograms as safe and sensible for normal nutrition.[13]

You cannot rely on even the lower figure from your diet. In 1981, I published a report in **Science** showing that selenium is deficient in the soils of most of Connecticut, Delaware, Illinois, Indiana, Massachusetts, New York, Ohio, Oregon, Pennsylvania, Rhode Island and the District of Columbia. If the soil is deficient, then so is the meat and the produce you eat, and therefore, so are you. The Colgan Institute routinely uses 200-400 micrograms of supplemental selenium in the form of organically bound l-selenomethionine, plus a smaller amount of the selenite form.

Glutathione Prevents Cancer

L-glutathione is one of your main endogenous (in the body) antioxidants. It is now thought to be a major cellular defense mechanism against carcinogens.[22] This discovery is vital to our understanding of cancer and other degenerative diseases, because glutathione levels decline with aging in mosquito, mouse and man.[23]

What happens if you can stop this decline? At the University of Louisville School of Medicine, Professor Calvin Lang and colleagues gave mosquitoes supplemental precursors of glutathione. Their glutathione levels shot up, and their lifespan was extended by a whopping 40%.[24]

A mosquito is not a good model for a man, but what about a

mouse? Drs. Jaime Miguel and Hans Weber of the Alexander Medical Foundation in San Carlos, CA, gave mice supplemental precursors of glutathione. Blood glutathione went up, and lifespan increased.[23]

There is also evidence that glutathione protects animals against **aflatoxin**, one of the most potent carcinogens.[25] No one knows the supplemental amount required to protect a man. But our extensive review of all the studies at the Colgan Institute, suggests that 250 mg per day of pre-formed L-glutathione may be adequate. To keep costs down, we use a mix of the expensive glutathione and its much cheaper precursor n-acetyl-cysteine.

Coenzyme Q10 Prevents Cancer

Your body can't make coenzyme Q10. It is derived from coenzyme Q, which occurs widely in foods, hence it's common name, ubiquinone (from ubiquitous).

Despite this abundance, the level of coenzyme Q10 declines in your body with age. This decline has now been traced to decline of an enzyme in the liver that converts Co Q to Co Q10.[26]

There are volumes of compelling evidence from animal and human research that you should maintain a high level of Co Q10 lifelong. In a typical study, Dr. Emile Bliznakov and colleagues at the New England Research Institute in Connecticut induced cancer in mice by injection of **dibenzpyrene**, the most potent carcinogen in tobacco. One group of mice was given a diet supplemented with Co Q10. The rest were not supplemented. Ten weeks later, every one of the unsupplemented mice had developed cancer. One quarter of the supplemented mice never developed cancer.[26]

Co Q10 has been a widely used nutrient in European and Japanese medicine since 1980. Nevertheless, amounts required to prevent cancer in man are still unknown. After reviewing all the literature, since 1985 the Colgan Institute has used supplements of 30-60 mg per day.

Antioxidants Protect Your Heart

How many people on a Friday night freeway will die of heart disease? Twenty percent? Thirty percent? The answer is *one in every two*. About half of all deaths in America are from coronary heart disease, most of them with advanced atherosclerosis.[27]

Most folk know (and hopefully care) that the typical American high-fat diet will raise cholesterol to high risk levels within a month, and that a low-fat diet will lower them. But only the best informed know that heart disease risk starts to rise at a cholesterol level of 168 mg/dl, not the 200 mg/dl now bandied about by the media.[28]

Most of us also know that regular exercise yields high levels of **high-density lipoproteins** (HDL), the "good" cholesterol that scrubs and vacuums excess cholesterol off the walls of your arteries.[29] But few people, and certainly not the popular media, seem aware of the last decade of research that uncovered the major mechanism by which atherosclerosis takes hold in the first place. The mechanism is oxidation. You can keep your cholesterol way down and your HDL high as a kite, but if you don't control oxidation, atherosclerosis will fill up your arteries like sockfuls of pudding.

In a simplified nutshell, it goes like this. Atherosclerosis starts with cells of your immune system called **monocytes**. These stick to the arterial wall, then pass through it and transform into scavenger cells called **macrophages** that gobble up wastes. That's all normal and dandy.

Problems arise when you subject the system to excess free radicals, such as you get from breathing polluted city air, or from eating pesticide contaminated food, or from many prescription drugs. Another potent source of oxidation is exercise.[30] Exercise uses up to 20 times more air than sitting in a chair and creates proportionately more free radicals.[1]

The excess free radicals begin to oxidize pesky little particles of cholesterol called **low-density lipoproteins** (LDL).[31] The immune system macrophages in the arterial walls recognize the oxidized LDLs as toxic to the body and gobble them up.[31,32] If you have excess LDLs, the macrophages soon become overstuffed with LDLs and break down into pathological cells called **foam cells**. These foam cells form the fatty streaks on the arterial walls that are the beginning of atherosclerosis.[33]

Antioxidant Protection

In its extraordinary wisdom, the Food and Drug Administration has decreed that manufacturers cannot make claims that antioxidants protect the heart. With all the evidence that they do just that, anyone with a cynical mind might well suspect political shenanigans. Certainly it would be disastrous for the medical industry if Americans began to live longer and remain healthy. Whatever the case, let's examine a little of the evidence from the pile of more than 100 studies now sitting at my right elbow, so you can decide for yourself. No one else is going to protect you.

Protection of LDL from oxidation depends on the fat-soluble antioxidants that can get inside the LDL particles, and the water soluble antioxidants that get into the fluids surrounding the LDL. You need some of both.

Best studied fat-soluble antioxidants are beta-carotene, vitamin E, and coenzyme Q10. Very recent evidence shows unequivocally that all three nutrients prevent oxidation of human LDL *in vitro* (in the test tube).[34,35,36]

Other studies show that the main water-soluble vitamin, vitamin C, acts synergistically to spare vitamin E stores by restoring used vitamin E to an active state.[31] More important, vitamin C prevents macrophages from absorbing LDL in the first place. In one new study by Drs. I. Jialal and S. Grundy at the University of Texas Medical Center, vitamin C prevented uptake of LDL by macrophages by 95%.[37] That makes vitamin C your first defense against atherosclerosis.

But, say the critics, that's all *in vitro*. What about in whole live humans? Well, this evidence is the cutting edge of science, so there are few human data. But I'm not waiting around until 2010 when the big clinical trials will be finished. I'll bet my more than 20 years of research the evidence reviewed above is on the money.

Just to sweeten the bet, preliminary findings from the University of Texas Medical Center, show that healthy volunteers supplemented with vitamin E are less subject to LDL oxidation than controls.[37] And monkeys supplemented with vitamin E show reversal of atherosclerosis.[38] Epidemiological studies also show that people with high intakes of beta-carotene, vitamin E, and vitamin C have a lower incidence of coronary heart disease.[39,40]

Finally, there are some results from the monster ongoing Physicians' Health Study in which thousands of American doctors are taking 50 mg of beta-carotene a day. A sub-group that had heart disease at the start of the study, already show a 44% reduction in heart attacks and death.[41] Examine the studies I have cited, and you may choose to join me in taking antioxidants to stay in good heart.

Antioxidants Inhibit Diabetes

Excess sugar levels in the blood of diabetics and pre-diabetics damage arteries, kidneys, eyes, and brain. One way to reduce this problem is to eat less sugar. But sugar is b-i-i-i-i-i-g business and billions are spent every year promoting and marketing sweets in every conceivable form.

The marketing is highly successful. As I write these words over lunch in Miracles Cafe in Cardiff-by-the-Sea, California, I am surrounded by fellow diners scarfing pastries, cakes and cookies by the oodle. We now consume half-a-pound of sugar per day for every man, woman and child in the nation.[42] No wonder many folk you pass in the street have crazed looks in their eyes.

Much of the sugar added to our food is hidden in label gobbledegook such as, "grape juice concentrate", and "sweetened with fruit juice", and "corn syrup". All these are simply refined liquid sugars. And our tardy health authorities have yet to advise the public that refined sugar is every bit as big a health risk as fat.

Their negligence has taken its toll. Pre-diabetes is now epidemic in America, with all its attendant problems of blindness, kidney failure, heart disease, and early death.[43]

We know now that diabetic damage from sugar occurs mainly by oxidation of fat molecules, to form toxic lipid peroxides. Numerous recent studies show that the antioxidant vitamin E can protect diabetic animals from this damage.[44] It works by complex mechanisms that also appear to neutralize sugar directly, in addition to reducing peroxide formation.

Looks like it works in human diabetics too. In the latest study, Dr. Guiseppe Paolisso, at the University of Naples in Italy, gave groups of diabetics and healthy controls 900 IU of vitamin E or a placebo for four months. Diabetics receiving the vitamin E showed significant reductions in blood sugar, thus reducing the potential for damage. They also showed significant increases in endogenous antioxidants, such as glutathione, indicating reduced pressure on the body's antioxidant defense system.[45] So even if you can't dodge all the sugar in your diet, antioxidants can save you from a lot of its damaging effects.

Antioxidants Boost Immunity

A pile of recent studies prove beyond doubt that antioxidants can inhibit, prevent or even cure hundreds of other diseases in addition to cancer, heart disease and diabetes. These include such widely diverse disorders as lung diseases,[46] cataracts, and macular degeneration of the eyes,[47] burns and other wounds,[48] anemia,[49] multiple different infections,[50] and degenerative diseases of the brain.[51]

How can such simple nutrients have such wide ranging benefits? Louis Pasteur, the father of modern medicine, gave the clue when on his deathbed. The drug-happy physicians surrounding him, received his final brilliant advice: ***"The key to medicine is host resistance"***. That's where antioxidants excel.

Antioxidants benefit your body not only by neutralizing free radicals directly, but also by increasing your resistance to all manner of toxins, bacteria, viruses, traumas, and degenerative diseases. They accomplish this amazing feat by boosting your immunity.

We began to appreciate this power of antioxidants only in the

1970s. Dr. Robert Tengerdy and colleagues at Colorado State University, discovered that supplementing animal diets with large amounts of vitamin E, protected them against various diseases and toxins deliberately introduced into their bodies. The basis of this protection was a big increase in immune strength, especially in strength of the lymphocyte responses.[52,53]

Control animals, whose diets contained the equivalent of an adequate amount of vitamin E for humans, according to the government RDAs, were not protected, and succumbed to disease after disease. By the 1980's, Tengerdy concluded from his research that to strengthen immunity may require at least *six times* the vitamin E that is deemed adequate for "normal" health.[54]

Other scientists obtained the same effect by using selenium, the antioxidant co-factor of vitamin E. Immune strength increased to *four times* the usual response.[55] Another study examined effects of selenium supplementation on a strain of mice called C3H. Because of an endemic virus throughout the strain, 80% of C3H mice develop mammary cancer. By long-term supplementation with selenium, mammary cancer was reduced to 10%.[56] Because it was acting against a virus, the effect of the selenium was not as a simple antioxidant. It was working as a complex booster of immune function.

Other studies show that antioxidant supplements given over long periods prevent the decline of animal immunity with aging.[57] And, even when animal immunity has declined with age, supplementary antioxidants can restore it, including a restoration of T-lymphocyte function.[58]

It works with human subjects too. In a typical study, Dr. Simin Meydani and colleagues at Tufts University Human Nutrition Research Center, supplemented healthy men and women over age 60 with 800 IU of vitamin E each day in a double-blind clinical trial. Most subjects receiving the vitamin E showed a 10% - 50% increase in immune strength, including increases in the production of lymphocytes.[59]

Even precursors of antioxidants can protect you. New studies show that protein from **whey** enhances immunity up to 500%. Other proteins have little effect.[60]

How does this happen? The main reason is that whey contains a much higher level of cysteine than most other proteins. Cysteine is the precursor of glutathione, one of the strongest antioxidants in your body. The studies show that glutathione levels increase rapidly in animals who are fed whey concentrate, and it is this increase that enhances immunity. So if you are using a protein drink for meal replacement or muscle building, make sure its first protein ingredient is whey protein concentrate.

I have given you only a brief sample of the evidence that daily supplementation with multiple antioxidants can provide amazing protection against multiple forms of disease and disorder. This protection is stronger by far than any physician, any hospital, any medicine, or any other health strategy known to man.

But it may be another decade before our government officially recommends antioxidants. So I cannot advise you to take them without risking prosecution. All I can do is present the evidence and let you decide for yourself. If you read the medical references given and choose wisely, then my purpose in writing this book to improve the health of America will be fulfilled.

Synergy of Antioxidants

One final all-important point. Do not use single antioxidants.

As with all other nutrients, antioxidants work properly only in *synergy* with each other. It is their multiple interactions that creates optimal protection for your body.

Let's look at an example to drive synergy home. Oral cancer is a good one. Chewing toxins such as tobacco, quickly causes oral leukoplakia, that is, pre-malignant lesions in the mouth and throat. Within a decade these lesions usually progress to cancer if left untreated, whether or not you give up the chew.

Vitamin E supplements can reverse leukoplakia in about 50% of cases. But vitamin E and beta-carotene combined can reverse leukoplakia in 65-75% of cases. [61,62]

Even the two antioxidants together do not provide optimal protection. Further studies deliberately induced oral cancer in animals, then tested vitamin E, beta-carotene, glutathione and vitamin C. Used singly, the antioxidants each provided some degree of cancer inhibition, glutathione and beta-carotene being the best. But, the combination of all four significantly reversed tumor growth. [63] So if you do choose to take antioxidants then ensure that the supplements contain at least the following major forms:

- Multiple forms of vitamin C, both as ascorbic acid and mineral ascorbates.

- Beta-carotene.

- Multiple forms of vitamin E, both as mixed tocopherols and d-alpha tocopheryl succinate.

- Two forms of selenium as selenomethione and as sodium selenite.

- L-glutathione.

- Zinc picolinate.

- Coenzyme Q10

I, my family and friends, and thousands of clients of the Colgan Institute worldwide have taken such a supplement for the last 21 years. We have found it to be the best health insurance there is.

Eat Your Veggies

That's not the end of the antioxidant story. The National Cancer Institute recommends eating fruit and vegetables as a cancer preventive, because they contain the antioxidants, vitamin C, vitamin E, and beta-carotene.[4] They are only partly right. Veggies do prevent cancer, but by far more powerful means than merely these three vitamins. Just when the medicine men thought they had a handle on antioxidants, researchers began to report from animal studies, that six other class of compounds in vegetables, prevent, and even reverse, cancer and a host of other diseases.

These health-giving natural compounds occur as some of the flavonoids in produce. Specifically they are **indoles, flavones, phenols, coumarins, isothiocyanates,** and **pycnogenols (procyanadins).** And much of their action is antioxidant too.[4,64]

Some folk seem surprised that so many important chemicals could hide for so long in simple vegetables. Don't be. Even the humble radish is a miracle of complexity far more intricate than the latest computer creation of man. I am indebted to my friend Dr. Richard Passwater for pointing out that known flavonoids in plants number over 20,000, and only 4,000 of them have yet been chemically analysed or tested.

In the six classes of new disease fighters, only about 100 of these compounds have been analysed and tested. Undoubtedly, there are many more we don't yet know about. But we do know they are powerful.

Brilliant researcher Dr. Gladys Block and colleagues at the University of California, Berkeley analyzed all 170 of the controlled studies to date on effects of fruit and vegetables on cancer. Some examples from their analysis:

Type of cancer	No. of studies showing protection
Lung cancer	24
Colo-rectal cancer	20
Stomach cancer	17
Esophageal cancer	15
Oral cancer	9
Cervical cancer	7

And on and on and on. We are now certain that the antioxidant flavonoids obtained by eating copious amounts of fruits and vegetables, can protect you against most types of cancer.[65] In fact, the realization is slowly dawning in nutrition science, that many of these compounds may be essential to maintain optimal health.

Tomatoes, carrots and strawberries all contain coumarins that prevent the formation of carcinogenic **nitroso compounds** in your intestines.[66] Green tea contains phenols, now shown in a pile of studies to inhibit stomach and esophageal cancer.[67,68] Cabbage, cauliflower, and broccoli contain indoles that prevent stomach and breast cancer.[69,70] My book **Prevent Cancer Now** covers the research on many other anti-cancer compounds in produce, occurring in everything from apricots to yams.[71]

Then there are the pycnogenols. You may see them called

catechins and **epicatechins** or **procyanadins**. They occur in produce too, but the most potent source is the coastal pine tree, *Pinus maritima*, that grows on the North Atlantic coasts of America and Canada. Used by native indians for thousands of years, pine bark pycnogenols have only now been re-discovered by modern science. They are powerful protectors against cancer and a variety of others diseases, including protecting the skin and organs from the usual damage of aging.[64]

Locked Into Nature

The antioxidant vitamins, C, E, and carotene in produce do help of course, but the amounts in many vegetables are so small that their effects are minor. Cabbage for example, supplies less that 2% of these vitamins in the American diet.[72] Yet this humble vegetable can stop breast cancer cold.

We know now how cabbage does the trick. To tell you I have to dip into a little biochemistry, but it provides a wonderful example of how our health is locked into compounds precisely designed by Nature to accomplish specific tasks in the human body.

Most breast cancer is linked to a deficit in estrogen metabolism.[73] The under-nourished female body can't de-activate its estrogen properly. It uses what is called the **estradiol 16-alpha hydroxylation** pathway, which leaves the hormone still active enough to cause cell transformation in the breast (and reproductive organs). Over years these cells gradually transform to cancer. The properly nourished female body, however, uses what is called the **estradiol 2-alpha hydroxylation** pathway, which neutralizes the hormone completely and never leads to breast cancer.[73]

To direct estrogen metabolism through the healthy pathway,

the body uses a chemical called **indole-3-carbinol**, one of the indoles that occurs in cruciferous vegetables. Green cabbage is an especially rich source. Both animal and human subjects given indole-3-carbinol show a 50-70% increase in healthy metabolism of estrogen, and a concomitant reduction in risk of cancer.[74]

Nature made all the locks and holds all the keys. Scientists are now realizing there are probably thousands of these natural compounds, most of them yet unknown, each with specific tasks to do in maintaining human flesh. The design of the human body is inextricably entwined with these substances, and, without them, your life is likely to be sad, painful, and short.

Even though the science for some of these compounds is now well established, the profit-motivated restrictions of our disease industry make it doubtful they will hit mainstream medicine any time soon. With breast and reproductive system cancers for example, we are in the ludicrous position that hospitals cannot use indole-3-carbinol to stop the disease, because it is not an approved drug. To get a good supply you have to eat cabbage.

Against the glittering backdrop of modern medicine's high-tech bells and whistles, a number of cancer hospitals are now effectively treating breast cancer with plain, old cabbage juice. H'mmm, that's just what Great-Grandma used to drink back in the days when breast cancer was a much rarer malady. Funny that.

Most Americans today don't eat their cabbage, or any other vegetable. Dr. Gladys Block has shown that the average intake is less than one serving per day of either fruit or vegetables (excluding potatoes and lettuce).[75] I hope you eat yours!

If you don't, can't or won't, the main effective flavonoids are now available in supplement pill form. But before you buy a particular brand make sure it contains all six classes listed above. In concert with the vitamin antioxidants, they are better health insurance than could ever be provided by the Tweedledum posturing on Capitol Hill.

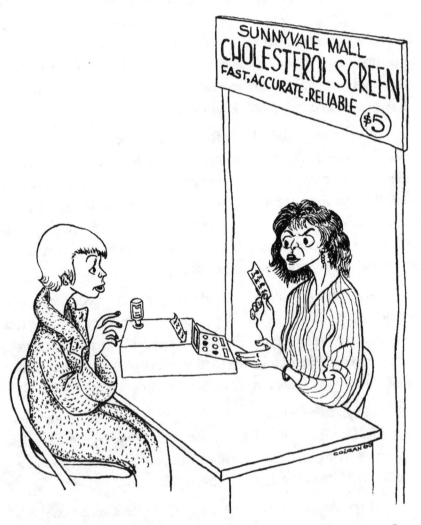

"Your cholesterol is 188 and you're going to meet a tall dark stranger."

Chapter 21

Good Fats, Bad Fats

Since March 1990, government health authorities have recommended that all Americans over age two should reduce their intake of saturated fats below 10% of daily calories, and their total intake of fats below 30% of daily calories. These recommendations were first proposed in the 1960s and, at that time, represented a fair approximation of the evidence that saturated fats and excessive total fats in the diet cause cardiovascular disease and certain cancers.

During the 25 years it took for the recommendations to wend their weary way through the ponderous committees of our health authorities, nutrition science made mighty advances. The 1960's advice is now obsolete. We know now that, *if you follow current government advice on fat intake you are likely to damage your body beyond repair*. That's putting it hot and heavy but, as you will see, the new evidence is irrefutable.

How Much Fat Do You Need?

Fat is your body's major fuel and some folk still believe you have to eat a lot of it to maintain energy. They are dead wrong. A slim man of 175 lbs who is only 10% bodyfat, carries 7% of that fat as a fuel store. This fat store weighs 5500 grams. At 9 calories per gram, it holds 49,500 calories, enough to run a hundred miles.

Contrast this fat store with his other major source of fuel, glycogen. At 4 calories per gram, his 450 grams of glycogen store holds only 1800 calories. Because your muscles cannot function without a minimum level of glycogen, the limit on energy is always glycogen, never fat.

So even a very slim person never runs out of fat.[1] To maintain a sufficient fat store, you need to eat hardly any. Between 10% and 15% of daily calories is ample. If your body ever needed any extra, it can easily convert proteins and carbohydrates into fat.

Chapter 20 shows how bodyfat is put on much more readily by eating fat than other foods. And current government advice that it is OK to eat 30% of daily calories as fat, encourages you to eat a lot of it. The result is waddling before us. Four in every ten adult Americans in the workforce are now overweight,[2] and we are getting fatter every decade.[3]

As you will see in Chapter 22, overwhelming evidence shows that even moderate overweight is a direct cause of many diseases, and increases risks of disability and death in almost all diseases.[4,5] With their current recommendations on fat intake, our health authorities are unwittingly making you sick.

Essential Fats

All fats are made of fatty acids, composed of a fat bit and an acid bit. Their chemical make-up is a carbon chain made of carbon and hydrogen atoms. Different fats have different length carbon chains. Short-chain fats such as butyric acid in butter have four carbons. Fish oils, and the long-chain fats that comprise most of your brain have 20 to 24 carbons.

In addition to the fat you use for fuel, your body requires many special fats. These serve as components of the cell membranes around every cell, and as components of your brain, inner ear, eyes, adrenal glands and sex organs.

Your body can make these special fats only if it gets the right raw materials in your diet. The right materials are two essential fats your body cannot make, **linoleic acid** and **alpha-linolenic acid**, both of which are long-chain (18 carbons). For optimum health, these two fats have to be provided by your diet. The body can transform them into every other kind of fat it needs.[6]

Unfortunately, essential fats are scarce in the average diet. The best source of linoleic and alpha-linolenic acids is **flax** or **linseed oil**. Other sources are **pumpkin seeds, walnuts, soybeans**, and **canola oil**. Dark green leaves of leaf vegetables also contain small amounts.[7] Good but expensive oil sources used in supplements are **blackcurrant seed oil, borage oil, evening primrose oil** and **fish oils**.

The fat content of common seed oils is shown in Table 9. This table applies only to cold-pressed, unprocessed oils that have not been hydrogenated. As you will see, when even the best oils are processed into margarine and cooking oils, they lose their healthful attributes.

Table 9: The percentage of fats in vegetable oils. The good, the bad, and the ugly.*

	Polyunsaturated Fats		Mono-	Saturated
	Linoleic Acid	α-Linolenic Acid	Unsaturated Fats	Fats
The Good Oils				
Flaxseed (linseed)	5	54	22	9
Pumpkin seed	45	15	32	8
Soybean	42	11	32	15
Walnut	50	5	29	16
Canola	26	8	57	9
Second Best				
Almond	17	-	68	15
Virgin Olive	12	-	72	16
Safflower	70	-	18	12
Sunflower	66	-	22	12
Corn	59	-	25	16
Sesame	45	-	45	13
Rice Bran	35	-	48	17
The Bad Oils				
Peanut	29	-	56	15
(Contains carcinogenic aflatoxin)				
Cottonseed	48	-	28	24
(May contain toxins)				
The Ugly Oils				
Palm	9	-	44	48
Palm kernel	2	-	18	80
Coconut	4	-	8	88

* These percentages hold only for fresh unprocessed, cold-pressed oils that have not been hydrogenated.

Source: The Colgan Institute, San Diego, CA.

Saturated Versus Unsaturated Fats

Saturated fats have all their carbon atoms "saturated" with hydrogen atoms. They have no empty hydrogen spaces to link up with the hydrogens of other molecules in your body. Consequently, they can be used by the body only for energy. Unsaturated fats have empty spaces where hydrogen atoms are missing. These spaces form special keys that can fit the locks of other molecules in your flesh.

Health authorities would have you believe that saturated fats come mainly from meats and raise cholesterol levels, and vegetable oils are unsaturated and keep cholesterol down. They are dead wrong!

It's true that meats, cheese, eggs, and milk are high in saturated fats. But so are **palm oil**, **palm kernel oil**, and especially **coconut oil** (See Table 9). In the mid '80s, I was one of a group of scientists who petitioned government to get these tropical vegetable oils out of our food - with some success. But many foods are still loaded with them. They raise cholesterol and low density lipoproteins (LDLs), and damage your health just as much as the greasiest fatback bacon.[8]

Also contrary to government health recommendations, recent evidence shows that not all saturated fats are bad. Careful controlled studies now indicate that **medium chain triglycerides (MCTs)**, which are saturated fats extracted from coconut oil, do not raise cholesterol. Neither does the saturated fat **stearic acid**.[9]

It gets worse. We know now that many of the so-called polyunsaturated fats approved by our health authorities, raise cholesterol over the moon because of what food processing has done to them. Remember, the good oils in Table 9 remain healthy only if they are unprocessed. Let's take a look at what happens to them on the way from the field to your table.

Cis Versus Trans Fats

Almost all natural fats occur in what is called a *cis* configuration. That is, the hydrogen atoms on the carbons are all on the same side of the molecule. Because of their slight electrical charge, the hydrogen atoms repel each other and put bends in the carbon chain like a series of overlapping horseshoes. These bends are the essential shape of the molecule, the key which fits the precise locks in your body that enable the special biological functions of fats to take place.

This essential cis configuration is destroyed by modern processing procedures, including heating, hydrogenation, bleaching, and deodorizing. These procedures are applied to almost all mass-produced fats and oils in America today. They change the healthy cis configuration into an unhealthy *trans* configuration. Chemically, the hydrogen atoms become rotated so that they lie on opposite sides of the fat molecule. The molecule then straightens out and loses its key shape that links with your cells in order to perform the biological functions of fats.

Your body is very adaptable. Even though the trans fats no longer fit its locks, it still has to try and use them for the essential functions of fats. In cell membranes for example, trans fats cause the membranes to leak, thereby disrupting cellular metabolism and permitting toxic substances to enter the cell. We know now that trans fats incorporated into cell membranes cause abnormal cell function that is implicated in both cardiovascular diseases and cancers.[10,11,12]

Government has disregarded this evidence, largely because of pressure from the oil-processing industry, and because the American diet contains only 3-4% of total calories as trans fats. Lobbyists persuaded politicians that disease effects would be negligible.[13] But recent animal studies have found gross cell abnormalities with diets of only 4.4% trans fats.[14]

Recent human studies published in the **New England Journal of Medicine** also show direct disease effects. Young, healthy males show elevated cholesterol levels and elevated low density lipoproteins (LDLs), if placed on a high trans fat diet for only three weeks. These elevations in cholesterol and LDLs are as high as those reached by feeding subjects a diet high in saturated fats from palm and palm kernel oils.[15] Current government health recommendations, which ignore the disease producing effects of trans fats, are directly promoting disease.

Identifying Trans Fats

All processed oils contain trans fats. The more solid the oil the higher the trans fat level. Liquid vegetable oils contain up to 6% trans fats and margarines and shortening up to 58%.[16,17]

You can identify trans fats in other foods by looking for the words "hydrogenated" or "partially hydrogenated" in the ingredients list. You will find these words on the labels of many breads, candies, baked goods, chocolate, frozen dinners, and processed meat products.[7] If you want the best of health, don't eat them.

The worst aspect of this trans fats nightmare is that the FDA, who are supposed to protect our food, remain 20 years behind the times. When the Center For Science In The Public Interest asked the FDA why the new 1994 regulations do not enable consumers to find out the level of trans fats in foods, the official replied, "We're exhausted from rule writing."[18] That's the sort of health protection that has made America sick.

The whole of Europe has had mandates against trans fats for some years. Many European foods now state specifically on the labels that they are made with cis fats, the healthy kind, even margarines. It will be years before we see it in the US. Meanwhile, buy and use only the good oils in Table 9. Especially buy and use organic flax oil. It will go a long way to protect your health.

Smart Fats

There are other important health reasons for using organic flax oil as a regular part of your nutrition. To understand them you have to know a little about what your body does with the two essential fats, linoleic acid and alpha-linolenic acid. Along the way I will show you why the two fish oils, eicosapentanoic acid (EPA) and docosahexanoic acid (DHA) are such powerful protection against disease. I will also tidy up common misconceptions about omega-3 and omega-6 fats. It's vital to know about these essential fats if you want to protect your health.

Figure 2 shows the sequence of special fats that your body makes from dietary essential fats. As you can see, linoleic acid from your diet is the start of the omega-6 sequence of fats. Like all fats in biochemistry, it has a descriptive number, cis 18:2 omega-6. Sounds complicated but it's really very simple. The number merely describes a series of bumps and hollows just like those on your car key.

Note first that the fats are in cis form. Biochemists know that only the cis form works in the human body. The first figure, in this case 18, describes the number of carbons that make up the length of the chain. The second figure, in this case 2, describes the number of hollows in the chain, that is, empty spaces for hydrogen atoms. These spaces create part of the key that fits the locks for specialized functions of fats in your body. The third figure, in this case 6, refers to the number of carbons along the chain where the first empty space

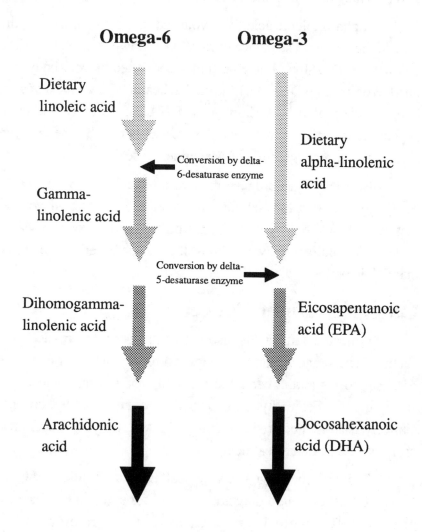

Figure 2. How the human body uses and converts the two essential fats.

occurs. This position creates the rest of the key.

Alpha-linolenic acid from your diet is cis 18:3 omega-3, the start of the omega-3 sequence of fats. Look down this sequence and you will see that alpha-linolenic acid is converted by your body first into EPA, then into DHA. DHA is vital to health because most of your brain is made of it.[19] A shortage of DHA causes inevitable brain degeneration, and is now believed by researchers to be one factor in America's current epidemic of Alzheimers disease.[19]

EPA and DHA are also the two omega-3 fats found in fish, especially oily fish like salmon, mackerel and sardines. If you eat these fish then you get your DHA preformed, saving your body a lot of work in making it. Now you know there's some truth to the notion that fish is brain food.

Omega-3s Fight Cancer

Omega-3 fatty acids also act in the body to produce vital chemical messengers called **prostaglandins**. Studies show that some of these prostaglandins can kill breast, lung and prostate cancer cells stone dead.[20] From this evidence, the **Journal of the National Cancer Institute** declared that omega-3 fats have "potential clinical usefulness" in cancer treatment.[20]

This evidence is vital to your health because studies show that omega-6 fats, although they are essential for some functions, also produce inflammatory prostaglandins that promote cancer growth.[21,22] Omega-3 fats keep this cancer effect of omega-6 fats under control.[20] For optimal resistance to cancer, you have to keep your intake of omega-3 fats dominant over omega-6.

Sadly, the American diet is very low in alpha-linolenic acid (omega-3), but high in linoleic acid (omega-6). As you can see from

Table 9, most vegetable oils have little or no omega-3 fats and a lot of omega-6 fats. The only common oil that contains a healthy balance is organic flaxseed. That's why it's so important for good health.

Omega-3s Stop Other Diseases

The benefits of omega-3 fats don't stop with cancer. I cannot cover the research here, but refer you to my book **Essential Fats: All You Need to Know About Fat Intake**. The evidence is impressive that a high intake of omega-3 fats (about a tablespoon of organic flaxseed oil per day) goes a long way to inhibit cardiovascular disease, adult-onset diabetes, some skin diseases, and rheumatoid arthritis.[23] Include omega-3s in your nutrition every day.

We are part of a universe filled with wonders just waiting for our wits to grow sharp enough to see them.

Michael Colgan

Chapter 22

Dieting Makes You Fatter

Slim is a national obession. Polls show that at any given time, over one-third of American women and one quarter of the men are trying to lose weight. In 1992, they spent $36 billion on it, and got almost nothing for their money.[1]

To put that huge sum in perspective, the total cost for all the 544,000 federal, state and local police officers in America and all the costs of law enforcement for 1993, came to 31.8 billion.[2]

So it is clear that Americans consider weight loss far more important than crime and personal safety. It is also clear that with such an enormous income, the weight-loss industry can and will do whatever it takes to maintain its customer base.

They are very busy at it. The last decade has witnessed an explosion of low-fat foods, no-cal drinks, meal replacements, appetite suppressants, weight loss clinics, diet books, gyms, chub clubs, and medical diets, all claiming they will take off the weight.

Almost all of it is marketing balderdash.

Sounds impossible that such a multi-billion dollar fraud goes on year after year without someone blowing the whistle. But it does. How do I know it's a fraud? Simple. Despite all the commercial weight-loss claims, celebrity endorsements, fat before and skinny after pics, and impossibly thin women in weeny bikinis, *the evidence is irrefutable that America is getting fatter every year.*[3,4]

Repeated National Health Examination Surveys since 1960 show that the average weight of American women aged 18-74 has increased by 4 lbs. The average weight of American men aged 18-74 has increased by 6 lbs.[5] Average heights remain almost unchanged, so there is no doubt that the nutrient poor American food supply is making us wider not taller, and that means fatter.

Data from the latest government study, released to the press by the National Institutes of Health on 17 March 1994, show that young adults are getting fattest of all. Males and females in the 25-30 age group are now 10 lbs heavier than the same age group was in 1986. And it's all useless blubber folks. The young hopes of the nation are bloating their way to premature oblivion.

Even by the government's generous standards of Body Mass Index, 32.6 million Americans are now classified as overweight.[5] Between ages 18 and 80, bodyfat levels typically increase from 15% to 35% in men and 20% to 40% in women.[6] As we will see, that's enough flab to cause every known major disease.

Exercise: What Exercise?

Hold on a minute, say my critics. What about the exercise craze? People are exercising more and putting on muscle, and that's good. I wish it were true. But when we look at the evidence, *the exercise craze that has supposedly swept America is a marketing myth*. It was cleverly designed by the weight-loss industry to induce you to buy home exercise equipment, health club memberships, "active" vacations and the like.

How do I know? Again, the evidence. After a 10-year study, the Centers For Disease Control in Atlanta report, that only 8% of adults aged 18-65 do any regular exercise (meaning 20 minutes or more of vigorous exercise three times or more per week).[7]

And, as those thousands of unused stair-steppers, exercycles, rebounders, cross-country trackers, and weight stacks that clutter garages from Nome to Miami attest, America is exercising less, not more. Couch potatoism is on the rise, even among the young and presumably vigorous. The latest survey of students in all 50 states shows that only 37% do any regular exercise. That's a huge *decline* from the 62% that exercised regularly in 1984.[8]

You have to face it folks. The detrimental effects of our denatured food, the marketing that keeps making us eat more of it, and the weight-loss industry, all conspire to make us fatter and sicker.

Sick Diets

Most popular diet books and weight-loss programs seem to be designed to distort your nutrition and promote disease. When you examine the methods used, they are so opposed to human physiology that a cynic might conclude, their main objective is to keep folk coming back repeatedly to highly profitable and terribly unsuccessful weight-loss schemes for the rest of their lives.

Analysis of twelve popular diets by Dr. Paul La Chance of Rutgers University shows that all of them rely on reducing your calories to the point where the amount of food eaten is seriously deficient in essential nutrients. The Beverly Hills Diet for example, provides one-quarter of the RDA for zinc, only one-third of the RDA for calcium, half the RDA for niacin and riboflavin, and deficient amounts of multiple other nutrients.[9] No one can be healthy on such regimens.

Muscle is the Engine

Low-calorie diets not only deprive your body of nutrients, they also cause devastating muscle loss. Nutrition scientists have known for decades that reducing calories to 800-1200 per day, which is below the body's essential energy requirement to maintain vital functions, causes you to cannibalize your own muscles for fuel. On these diets, muscle provides up to 45% of the energy deficit.[10]

If the deficit in essential energy requirement is 500 calories per day, then up to 225 calories will come from muscle breakdown. At 4 calories per gram that's 56 grams or 2 ounces. In only four weeks on such a diet, you can lose 3½ lbs of vital muscle.

Why is muscle so important? Any college physiology text will tell you that the adipose cells that store your bodyfat have little metabolic activity. They burn very few calories.[9] Fat sits like sausages, deadweight, until it is used for fuel. Muscle is different. It is always in motion. Opposing muscles are in constant dynamic tension to hold up your skeleton and enable you to do every movement you make.

But much more than that, *muscle is the engine of your body* where almost all your energy is created by burning of fats, carbohydrates, and proteins in the mitochondria (furnaces) of each and every muscle cell. Studies show that even an ounce of muscle lost, lowers your basal metabolic rate of fuel consumption, and reduces your ability to burn bodyfat.[11,12] So all diets that are below the essential energy requirement of your body are a guaranteed recipe for failure.

"Oh no! Not that dreadful tune again!"

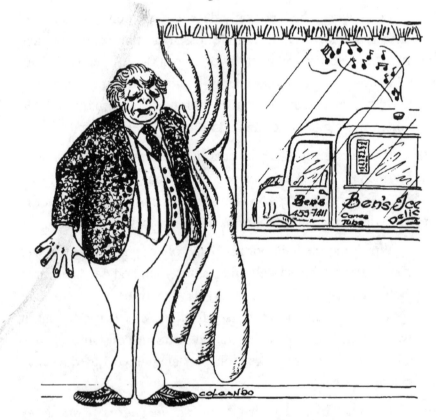

That Pesky Fat Storage Enzyme

Lately we have been assailed by a slew of the most weird and wonderful diet concoctions. Liquid meals, fiber bars, cellulose cakes, featherlight cereals, and sinless desserts, all pumping as much air as they can into as few calories as possible.

The weight-loss industry continues to push these low-cal confections for two reasons. First, they know that low-calorie diets cause rapid loss of both muscle and fat. In these days of instant mashed potatoes, while-you-wait spectacles, and total makeovers in sixty minutes or less, rapid effects are essential to continued sales. The average consumer doesn't know (or presumably care) that they are losing muscle along with the fat. All they want is weight off now.

The second commercial hook known to everyone in the business, is that rapid fat loss means guaranteed fat regain, setting up the customer for that essential repeat business. The physiology of it all has been known for fifty years. Rapid fat loss alerts your body's potent defenses of its energy reserve. It immediately increases the quantity and activity of an enzyme called **lipoprotein lipase**, its main mechanism for collecting digested fat from your bloodstream and stuffing it into fat cells.[13]

So lipoprotein lipase starts grabbing every molecule of fat, even stopping your body using it for energy. You have to burn even more muscle to make up the deficit. But muscle is harder and dirtier for the body to burn than fat (after all it is your basic structure). So your metabolism slows down, immediately reducing your ability to burn fat. You also get a build-up of toxic wastes from burning proteins, that makes you sick and cranky into the bargain. This activity does nothing to curb your appetite.[14] So you also grow progressively more ravenous.

It gets worse. When you can't stand the discomfort any longer and succumb to real food, lipoprotein lipase has become so efficient that you can regain six weeks of painful fat loss in almost as many days.

The big problem is, you don't regain any of the lost muscle. So the net result of the diet is no change in bodyfat but a big loss of muscle. This loss of part of your engine, reduces your ability to burn the fat you have, and sets you up for further fat gain.

Low-calorie diets cause so much muscle loss, that overweight people who use them repeatedly, train their bodies into **permanent** obesity. They have so little muscle left to burn fuel, that they have to eke out existence on 1000 calories a day, all the time. Otherwise they plump up like the Michelin Man.

We all know these sad, tired, overweight folk who eat like birds but never lose an ounce. Apart from a few unfortunates with genetic obesity, they are victims of the Great American Weight Loss Fraud. Don't become one of them.

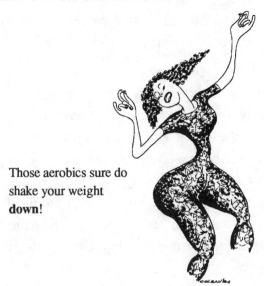

Those aerobics sure do shake your weight **down!**

The Bad And The Bogus

Don't get caught by the slimming aids scam either. A zillion miracle weight-loss products lurk round every corner to trap the desperate dieter. The shiny packages, well-known company names, and Madison Avenue gibberish on the labels all scream legitmacy, and promise slim Nirvana. Almost all of them are bogus.

How can I be so sure? When you ignore the labels and marketing hype and examine the evidence, they simply don't work.

Anti-cellulite creams for example, are sold by most top cosmetics houses. Dr. Peter Fodor, president of the Lipoplasty Society explains the simple physiology. You cannot remove a molecule of fat **under** the skin with creams or lotions applied on top of the skin, unless they contain a drug that penetrates the dermis to reach the fat underneath.[15] *All* skin-penetrating drugs of any efficacy are controlled prescription substances. So they cannot be used in over-the-counter cosmetics. So all the cellulite creams together cannot shift a single fatty ounce.[16]

What about the new fat-busting creams containing the asthma drug **aminophyline** or similar drugs, that claim to reduce fat on the thighs? These bogus products arose from equally bogus tabloid reports of a paper given at a 1993 meeting of the American Association for the Study of Obesity. Preliminary experiments showed that women lost an inch in thigh circumference after five weeks of vigorously rubbing in the cream every day. You can get similar effects by vigorously rubbing cream cheese on your thighs, because massage temporarily reduces thigh water content.

Even Dr. Bruce Frome who holds the license for the aminophyline cream used in the study, admits that, "within 3-7 days of non-use, the results disappear". Sounds like water not fat doesn't it. Don't waste your money.

More Bogus Supplements

Similarly ineffective are fiber pills because the amount of fiber per pill is negligible. Grapefruit pills don't work either because the amount of the active substance, **naringenin** is negligible. Herbal teas are mainly diuretic, so cause only temporary water loss. Artificial sweeteners do not curb appetite. So you tend to eat more calories from other foods than the calories saved by avoiding sugar.[16]

Bulking agents and starch blockers that are supposed to reduce food digestion, such as guar gum, glucomannan, and spirulena, don't work. Cellulose (wood fiber) used in weight-loss snacks gives you terrible intestinal problems. False fats only encourage you to eat fat. Intestinal peptides are destroyed by digestion.[16]

The list goes on *ad nauseum* down to rubber sweat suits, seaweed wraps and electronic muscle stimulators. If you believe any of them then Lord help you, because you are likely to end up fatter than Miss Piggy.

Commercial Diets Inneffective

If it sounds too incredible that government would permit this fraud to continue, then let me hammer home the lesson with the latest and strongest evidence. You might expect that the best low-calorie diets would be the expensive, medically supervised programs, such as Optifast and Medifast, that include professional behavior therapy and extended counselling, and are run through hospitals and medical facilities. They don't work.

In 1988 San Diego State University studied over 200 people who had lost an average of 84% of their excess weight on such medically supervised diets. Within three years subjects had regained 60-80% of the pudge.[17]

Results of this and similar studies finally stirred the slumbering National Institutes of Health and FDA. In 1992 they mounted a nationwide investigation by a panel of thirteen of the country's top experts on overweight, headed by Dr. Suzanne Fletcher, editor of the respected **Annals of Internal Medicine**. All the big diet programs and weight-loss centers submitted their records for analysis. The panel's report concluded that there is no evidence that *any* popular weight-loss program has much chance for long-term success. They further concluded that the public is being presented with reports of the few individual successes, and not being told that most people who take the programs either drop out before completing them, or regain most or all of the weight lost.[18]

The Federal Trade Commission instructed weight-loss companies, including the medically supervised programs, to stop making overblown claims. This slap on the wrist has changed the language of the ads into meaningless jingles, but the flim-flam continues. If you want to get fatter, join up today!

Public belief in TV diet ads is a perfect example of the way in which vain desires can be manipulated to produce the same mass suspension of reason that gave us Hitler, Saddam Hussein, and ethnic cleansing.

Michael Colgan
Nutrition Lectures, 1994

Chapter 23

Overweight Is Illness

Calling fat folk sick may raise some hackles in our cringing new era of political correctness. But in cold reality, people of color are still financially deprived, waitpersons still wait, and ecological executives still hump the garbage. A spade is still a spade, and the "gravitationally challenged" still bear America's heaviest health burden.

Bodyfat Breeds Heart Disease

Let's examine the fat/sick link. The Framingham Heart Study has been going on now for over three decades. It's America's best. Successive follow-ups over 26 years, show that weight gain after adulthood causes a huge increase in risk of all types of cardiovascular disease.[1]

It doesn't have to be much pudge. Even a 10% increase above ideal weight causes a 6-7% increase in blood pressure. That's only 15 lbs extra on a 150 lb person. And losing that extra weight causes an immediate drop in blood pressure of 10-11%.[2] So there's no doubt that the bodyfat was causing the illness.

The seriously overweight folk are in dire straights. Women for example, carrying 50-60 lbs of extra padding are **700%** more likely to develop hypertension.[2]

...And Diabetes

Serious overweight also causes rapid diabetes. Both men and women carrying 60 lbs. extra or more, are **3000%** more likely to develop diabetes. Even moderate overweight increases your risk of diabetes by about 100%.[3]

...Cancer Too

Cancer also loves bodyfat. The American Cancer Society did a massive 20-year study involving over a million Americans in 25 different states. Results showed that men who are 40% overweight, have higher rates of prostate cancer, colon cancer and rectal cancer. Women who are 40% or more overweight, have higher rates of breast cancer, ovarian cancer, uterine cancer, gall bladder cancer, cervical cancer, and endometrial cancer.[4] Corpulent is sick indeed.

...And All The Rest

I can cover only a fraction of the fat/sick studies because overweight is a big cause of almost all diseases. Even moderate fatness damages the immune system, reducing your resistance to everything.[5] Being overweight going into surgery, for example, increases your risk of post-operative infections by up to 700%.[6] And, giving the lie to those "healthy fat cheeks" of childhood, studies show that fat babies get twice as many infections as slim babies.[7]

Just A Little Happy Fat

Folk who are only moderately overweight show typical defensive reactions to the evidence that fat is sick. They suck in their stomachs and laugh, "This is just happy fat". Or they slap a plump thigh and exclaim, "God made me this way, healthy and comfortable".

The latest study shows that even the mildly chunky die young. At the Harvard School of Public Health, Dr. I-Min Lee and colleagues tracked 19,297 healthy Harvard men who graduated between 1916 and 1950. Smokers were excluded as unacceptable health risks.

By 1988, 4370 of the men had died - mostly chunky. The less the men weighed throughout life, the lower their risk of death. Men who were 20% below the average for Americans of comparable age and height had the best expectation of long and healthy lives.[8]

With 32.6 million Americans classified as overweight and about another 40 million on the way, bodyfat is by far our worst health risk. It causes more illness than all the environmental and nutrition problems, than smoking, alcohol and all other drugs put together. It's infinitely worse than over-publicized AIDS.

Yet, to the ignorant, overweight is little more than a good butt for humor. It is sort of comical that Americans waddle enough fat around to feed the whole of starving Africa, and would gladly pay the shipping, but the disease it causes is no joke.

Don't despair. The next chapter gives you all the tools you need to reshape your body lean for life.

Obesity is wide spread.
Michael Colgan

Chapter 24

Lean
For Life

Overweight is your greatest health risk, so this is the most important chapter in the book. But it's not complicated. Once you know how the human body works, becoming lean for life is easy as momma's apple pie.

Most folk who come to the Colgan Institute object, "But I've tried every which way, and look at me". We usually find they have tried commercial weight-loss systems, or fad diets, or bogus slimming aids, which as we have seen, only set you up to become fatter.

By using this book you save yourself all that aggravation. You also save all the cost of professional visits, psychological counselling, or complex behavior therapy. In fact, most such intervention is detrimental. In 1992, the National Institutes of Health expert panel on weight loss, showed that behavior therapy and counselling, get *worse* long-term results than folk simply losing weight by themselves.[1] All you need are the principles given here. Follow them step-by-step and you will grow leaner than your wildest dreams.

Lose Fat Slow, Slow, Slow

It's obvious that folk differ widely in their inborn tendencies to store fat. But some researchers have overblown the obvious to claim that each person is designed to be healthy only at a certain fat level, and that the body will always revert to that level.[2] They are dead wrong.

The amount of fat you carry is not ordained by your genes. It is caused by what you eat and what you do. Recent science has shown that neither the number of fat cells nor their size is genetically fixed.[3] Bodyfat is much more dependent on lifestyle.

Your body has no internal reference for a permanent level of fat, only for a habitual level. When you remain at a particular level of fat for a year or more, your body develops all the adipose cells, capillaries, enzyme counts, peripheral nerves, hormone levels, and connective tissue to support it. It comes to recognize that level of fat as self and will defend it vigorously. That is your **fatpoint**.

The body constantly monitors its fatpoint with hormonal messengers, such as **glycerol**, which warn the brain to take defensive action if even one pound is suddenly used for fuel. So usual forms of dieting can't possibly work. As we have seen earlier, by slowing metabolism, increasing fat storage, and increasing appetite, your body's fatpoint defenses will defeat you every time.

Then how can you beat it? Easy. Reliable studies show that it takes years of overeating to grow fat.[4] Bodyfat typically creeps on by only an ounce or so per day, a pound every two or three weeks. In a year you are 20 lbs over. In 3-4 years you gain 60 lbs of flab.

Your body shifts its habitual fatpoint *up* very slowly. To shift it *down*, you have to operate the same way, very slowly. Otherwise the body will cannibalize your muscle, excite your fat storage enzyme, and boost your appetite to ravenous.

The first trick is to reduce your total daily calories by **no more than 20%**. That's 400 calories off a 2000 calorie diet. That's 2800 calories or 0.8 lbs of fat per week. Because of increases in body efficiency, you will not lose 0.8 lbs of fat but only about half a pound. That's the most you can lose without triggering body defenses.
Step 1: Lose no more than half-a-pound of fat per week.

Ditch The Scales

Scale weight varies day-to-day by up to five pounds depending on body water and food residue. To ensure that you are losing fat and not muscle or water, stop weighing and throw your scales away. Instead, get your body composition measured once a month, including fat weight, lean weight and body water.

Don't do it more frequently, because the drop in fat levels on an average size person is only about 1% per month. That is about the limit of accuracy of any measure of body composition. So more frequent measures than once a month, confuses instrument error with changes in bodyfat.

After testing dozens of professional systems, the Colgan Institute recommends only two, underwater weighing, and near infrared inductance using the Futrex 5000 device. Go to the same facility each time, because systems are all calibrated differently.

A newly available alternative is inexpensive skin-fold calipers for self-use at home. These calipers have a tension device on them to ensure you get the same pressure on the fat each time you measure. Provided you take the measurements in exactly the same spots on each occasion, we have found them very reliable.
Step 2: Measure your bodyfat once a month.

Fat Calories Are Fatter

The calories you cut from your diet have to be the right calories. First and most important is calories from *all* kinds of fat. Contrary to the calorie-counting strategies of much of the weight-loss industry, we now know that fat calories are fatter.

When excess carbohydrate or protein are eaten, the body makes complex metabolic adjustments to promote glycogen storage in muscle, and increase the use of protein or sugar for fuel.[5] It also has to use a lot of energy to convert these foods to bodyfat. Hence you have to eat a bigger excess of carbs and protein than you do of fat before they end up on your hips. But when excess fat is eaten, metabolism remains unchanged. Virtually all the excess is promptly layered onto all the wrong places.[6]

Now you know why calorie counting doesn't work. Numerous recent studies show that you put on much more bodyfat by eating fat, than by eating the *same number of calories* from carbohydrate or protein.[7,8,9]

In a typical experiement, Dr. Wayne Miller and colleagues at the University of Illinois, gave one group of rats a diet containing 42% fat. They gave a second group a low-fat diet of rat chow. Both groups ate as much as desired.

Over 60 weeks, both groups ate almost exactly the same number of calories (36,000 per rat). Common beliefs in the weight-loss industry would predict that both groups would be equally fat. No way. Only the high-fat group were plump, over 21% fatter than the low-fat group.[10] Many such studies now show that fat calories pack on more bodyfat than calories from any other food.

Step 3: Eat a low, low-fat diet.

How Much Fat?

The FDA labelling laws that came into effect on 9 May 1994 make it much easier for consumers to assess the fats in food. Fat content is now given by calories. All you have to do is compare the total calories per serving with the fat calories.

The new Nutrition Facts label is shown in Figure 3. It has to appear on all packaged food. Don't buy foods without it. They are either illegal or have lain too long on the store shelf.

Look at the line near the top showing calories. Divide the total calories (in this case 90) by the calories from fat (in this case 30). If the answer is less than 5 (in this case it is 3), don't buy the food.

An answer of 5 or more means that the food gets 20% or less of its calories from fat. You should not eat any food more fatty. In a diet of 2000 calories, that's a maximum of 400 fat calories. At 9 calories a gram, that's 44 grams of total fat per day. One double cheeseburger can contain 60 grams of fat, greasy evidence for a major source of America's health problems.

Step 4: Do not eat foods containing more than 20% fat calories.

Hidden Fats

Many failed dieters believe they are following healthy low-fat nutrition, when in fact they are being fooled into fatness by false food labelling. Many apparently dry foods like cookies, baked goods, crackers and chips, are higher in fat than ice-cream. Even low-fat milk is really high fat.

How does low-fat milk get away with its name? By jiggery-pokery lobbying power, the dairy industry got an exemption from the new labels. Nevertheless, an 8 oz glass of low-fat milk (2%) serves

Nutrition Facts

Serving Size 1/2 cup (114g)
Servings Per Container 4

Amount Per Serving

Calories 90   Calories from Fat 30

	% Daily Value*
Total Fat 3g	**5%**
Saturated Fat 0g	**0%**
Cholesterol 0mg	**0%**
Sodium 300mg	**13%**
Total Carbohydrate 13g	**4%**
Dietary Fiber 3g	**12%**
Sugars 3g	
Protein 3g	

Vitamin A	80% •	Vitamin C	60%
Calcium	4% •	Iron	4%

* Percent Daily Values are based on a 2,000 calorie diet. Your daily values may be higher or lower depending on your calorie needs:

	Calories	2,000	2,500
Total Fat	Less than	65g	80g
Sat Fat	Less than	20g	25g
Cholesterol	Less than	300mg	300mg
Sodium	Less than	2400mg	2400mg
Total Carbohydrate		300g	375g
Fiber		25g	30g

Calories per gram:
Fat 9   •   Carbohydrates 4   •   Protein 4

Figure 3. The new food label, now mandatory on packaged foods since May 1994.

you a hefty one-third of its calories from fat.

Food industry lawyers have filed exemption claims for all kinds of foods. And thousands of copywriters are busily writing new loopholes round the laws. So if you want to avoid hidden fats, don't trust anything on food labels except the **Nutrition Facts** panel. To be legal that has to be accurate.

Especially beware the slew of "reduced fat" products. Under the label laws "reduced fat" means 25% less fat than the original product. Oreo cookies for example are 44% fat calories. The new Reduced Fat Oreos are legal, but still load you with one-third of their calories as fat.

So it goes with everything from reduced fat bologna, which can still be 60% fat, to "light" and "lite" variants of foods, that have to be one-third less fat than the original, but can still be 40-50% fat. *Step 5: Trust only the Nutrition Facts panel on food labels.*

Sugar: Brown, White, Hidden, and Deadly

The second edible to cut down in your diet is simple sugars. Chocolate, candy, cookies and table sugar are obvious. But raw sugar, brown sugar, refined honey, high-fructose corn syrup, fruit juice concentrates, date sugar, and turbinado sugar are just as bad.

So are fruit juices. Ounce for ounce, orange juice contains more sugar than Coca Cola. And sodas in general contain up to 10 teaspoons of sugar per serving.

Why does sugar pile on bodyfat? Because its quick absorption into your bloodstream causes an excess insulin burst from the pancreas. On reaching your liver, excess insulin, which is toxic, is converted to neutral triglycerides. Triglycerides are exactly the form of fats that are stored in all your adipose cells.

So sugar not only loads you with excess calories that eventually turn to fat, but also causes the body to make even more fat from its own insulin.

Replace as much of the simple sugars in your diet as you can with complex carbohydrates. Essentially these are whole grains and vegetables, as little processed as possible.

Step 6: Cut the sugar, eat complex carbohydrates instead.

Regular Meals

A typical home handyman way to lose weight is to skip meals. Many folk skip breakfast or have just a piece of fruit for lunch, in the false belief it will carve off the chub. Sorry to disappoint you. Such strategies *increase* bodyfat because they result in yo-yo insulin bursts as soon as you eat again. The excess insulin that is turned into fat can easily compensate for the skipped meal. What you are doing is simply converting more of your body into fat.

One big secret of lean for life is to keep your insulin output even all day long. I cover all the evidence in my book **Optimum Sports Nutrition**.[14] To keep insulin steady never miss meals. In fact, for optimum fat loss, reduce the size of each meal and get into the habit of eating five small meals per day.

Step 7: Don't skip meals. Eat five small meals per day.

No Popular Diets

As we saw earlier almost all popular diets are deficient in essential nutrients. It may be tempting to eat only grapefruit, or only bananas and milk, or only salads, to name three recent diets, but they are all nutrient poor. The net result is to give you nutrient deficiencies that turn up your appetite to unstoppable, making you fatter and sicker.

Instead of this dieting insanity, follow the Eating Right Pyramid in Chapter 2 and eat a wide variety of foods.
Step 8: Avoid all fad diets.

Take Nutrient Supplements

As we have seen throughout this book, most of our food has become deficient in many vitamins and minerals. Your body registers these deficiencies, and turns up your appetite to making you eat more to supply the missing nutrients.

Because the nutrients are scarce in our food, you have to eat far too many calories to provide them. If even one nutrient remains deficient, your body will continue asking for it via your appetite. A single nutrient deficiency is enough to make you fat as a hog.

The simplest answer to this problem is to take a complete multi-vitamin supplement plus a complete multi-mineral supplement every day. These supplements provide an important regulator to the appetite, and naturally curb your desire to eat.

Table 10 shows the amounts and forms of each nutrient in supplements used by the Colgan Institute that will provide complete vitamin and mineral nutrition.
Step 9: Take a high-quality mutli-vitamin and multi-mineral supplement every day.

Chromium Reduces Fat

The US National Academy of Sciences believed that chromium was great for car bumpers but useless for human nutrition. Then Dr. Walter Mertz of the USDA Human Nutrition Research Center in Beltsville, MD, showed that chromium is essential for your

Table 10: Multi-vitamin/mineral basic formula.

Fat Soluble Vitamins

Beta-carotene	12,500 IU	A (retinol)	7,500 IU
D_3 (Cholecalciferol)	400 IU	E (d-alpha tocopherol)	400 IU
K (phylloquinone)	75 mcg		

Water Soluble Vitamins

B_1 (thiamin)	50 mg	B_2 (riboflavin)	45 mg
B_3 (niacin)	50 mg	B_3 (niacinamide)	80 mg
B_5 (pantothenic acid)	150 mg	B_6 (pyrdioxine)	50 mg
B_{12} (cobalamin)	100 mcg	Biotin	500 mcg
Folic acid	400 mcg	C (ascorbic acid)	250 mg
C (calcium ascorbate)	250 mg	C (ascorbyl palmitate)	150 mg
C (magnesium ascorbate)	100 mg		

Essential Fatty Acids

Linoleic acid	150 mg	Alpha-linolenic acid	250 mg
Gamma-linolenic acid	25 mg		

Lipogenics

Phosphatidyl choline	200 mg	Inositol	200 mg

Accessory Nutrients

Coenzyme Q10	30 mg	Citrus bioflavonoids	350 mg
Para-amino-benzoic acid (PABA)	35 mg		

Minerals*

Calcium (carbonate)	800 mg	Magnesium (aspartate)	600 mg
Potassium (aspartate)	100 mg	Iron (picolinate)	10 mg
Zinc (picolinate)	15 mg	Manganese (gluconate)	5 mg
Boron (aspartate)	3 mg	Copper (gluconate)	500 mcg
Chromium (picolinate)	200 mcg	Iodine (potassium iodide)	100 mcg
Molybdenum (trioxide)	60 mcg	Selenium (selenomethionine)	200 mcg

* Mineral amounts given are elemental, that is actual amounts of the element itself, not the amounts of the compound in which the element is provided. For example, calcium carbonate is only 40% calcium. So to provide 800 mg of calcium, you require 2,000 mg of calcium carbonate.

Source: Colgan Institute, San Diego, CA.

body to use insulin. That discovery changed official policy in a hurry. Now the latest **RDA handbook** recommends 50-200 mcg of chromium per day to maintain insulin metabolism.[11]

Because of the huge incidence of diabetes in America, folk are well aware that insulin enables the body to deal with sugar. But usually they don't know that insulin also controls fat and muscle.[12]

Problem is, virtually none of us gets even the lower recommended level of chromium in our degraded food. Drs. Richard Anderson and Adrienne Kozlovsky showed recently that 90% of the self-selected diets of Americans contain less than 50 mcg of chromium per day. Average chromium intake is only 29 mcg.[13] With that sort of nutrition, your insulin metabolism is barely limping along, and the bodyfat piles on.

Fortunately, a new form of chromium, **chromium picolinate** can help. Since its development by Dr. Gary Evans for the US government in the early '80s, chromium picolinate has been a boon. In my book **Optimum Sports Nutrition**, I review more than 20 studies showing that it improves insulin metabolism, reduces bodyfat, and increases muscle mass.[14]

There are plenty of studies showing that chromium picolinate reduces bodyfat in humans, but I like best the studies on pigs. Pigs have similar insulin metabolism to men, and, like men, tend to overeat and put on fat. But, unlike men, pigs can't cheat. They don't even know they are in a study, or that tasteless chromium picolinate has been added to their feed. They just belly up to the trough and gobble.

In a typical series of studies at the Department of Animal Science of Louisiana State University in Baton Rouge, pigs fed chromium picolinate increased their lean mass by 7% and reduced their bodyfat by 21%. That's a much healthier animal.[14]

Your daily multi-mineral supplement should contain 200 mcg of chromium picolinate. For a sedentary person of normal weight, that is probably sufficient. But for fat loss, the Colgan Institute uses an additional 200-600 mcg of chromium picolinate per day, in conjunction with exercise. This amount allows not only for the increased chromium required to metabolize fat, but also for the increased use of chromium by exercise.[14]

Even 800 mcg of chromium picolinate is completely innocuous. But don't use any other form of chromium at this level. Hexavalent chromium or chromate, for example, is highly toxic.[11]
Step 10: Use a chromium picolinate supplement every day.

Essential Fat To Lose Bodyfat

There is more to insulin metabolism than chromium. Dr. Leonard Storlien and colleagues at the Garvin Institute for Medical Research in Australia, were the first to show that the omega-3 fats found in fish oils, and also made by your body from the alpha-linolenic acid in flax oil, improve insulin efficiency in using carbohydrates and fats for fuel.[21]

As we saw in Chapter 21, most Americans are deficient in omega-3s. To combat bodyfat make sure that you get yours. At the Colgan Institute we use a tablespoon of organic flax oil or the equivalent in capsules.
Step 11: Take a flax oil essential fatty acid supplement every day.

Carnitine Moves Fat

Bodyfat is stored in adipose cells, but is burned for energy only in the mitochondria (furnaces) of muscle cells. To get from the adipose cells to the muscle cells, fat is carried by a nutrient called **l-carnitine**.[16]

The higher the level of l-carnitine in muscle, the more bodyfat is transported and burned. Studies show that supplements of l-carnitine raise muscle carnitine levels.[17] Therefore they also help you to lose bodyfat.

Your body makes l-carnitine. But, if you are overweight and yet don't eat a lot, it probably doesn't make enough for optimum use of fat for fuel. To promote fat loss, the Colgan Institute uses 2-4 grams per day of l-carnitine in conjunction with exercise.

If you decide to use it, make sure you get l-carnitine which is expensive. Racemic carnitine or dl-carnitine is cheap and toxic and interferes with l-carnitine metabolism, so actually *increases* bodyfat.[18] If anyone offers you carnitine cheap, smile and politely refuse. You know better.

Step 12: Use an l-carnitine supplement every day.

Fiber Fights Fat

High-fiber diets (30-50 grams per day) are not only great disease preventers, but also create slow, even food absorption from your intestines. This process helps keep your insulin level steady and also promotes use of the food for energy rather than for deposition as bodyfat.[19]

But most of us don't get enough fiber. Figures from the National Cancer Institute show that average American consumption of fiber is only 10-20 grams per day.[20] That low intake promotes a lot of disease and puts on a lot of bodyfat. NCI recommends 25-35 grams of fiber per day to prevent colon and rectal cancer.[20] For that reason alone fiber is essential.

For efficient control of bodyfat, the Colgan Institute recommends 40-50 grams of mixed fibers per day. Table 11 gives you food portions of common foods that each provide 10 grams of fiber. The rest is up to you.

Step 13: Eat 40 grams of mixed fibers every day.

Exercise Is Essential

Dr. Peter Wood of Stanford University has shown repeatedly that exercise is more important than food intake in regulating bodyfat. Regular exercisers eat a lot more than sedentary people but are a lot slimmer.

And if you get a plump person to do the right exercise at the right time, they can increase their caloric intake way *above* the amount used by the exercise and still lose a lot of fat.[22]

The key is to do the right exercise. The usual advice in the weight-loss industry is aerobics and more aerobics, and the more intense the better. Wrong! Wrong! Wrong!

Aerobic exercises that raise your heart rate above about 120 beats a minute, including running, rowing, swimming, cycling, and many of the fancy aerobics classes in health clubs, all strip off muscle almost as much as they strip off fat. And you have already learned what muscle loss does: it reduces your ability to burn fat, and sets you up to become fatter.

Remember, *muscle is the engine in which bodyfat is burned*. You should do everything you can to maintain it lifelong. Mild aerobics, such as walking is good exercise for many health reasons. It also burns some fat and will not burn muscle. But far and away the best exercise for fat control, is wide-variety, high-repetition resistance training, using weights or machines. By exercising muscles all over

Table 11: Fiber "10".

	Each item contains 10 grams of dietary fiber. Aim for 40-50 grams per day.
Grains	½ cup all bran 1 cup rolled oats 1 cup whole grain cereal 2 cobs sweet corn 3 slices whole rye bread 3 cups puffed wheat 4 oz. bag popcorn
Vegetables	½ cup mixed beans, lentils ½ cup peas 1 cup peanuts 2 cups soybeans 2 cups steamed vegetables 4 servings mixed salad 4 carrots
Fruits	3 pears 3 bananas 4 peaches 4 oz. blueberries 5 apples 6 oranges 6 dried pear halves 10 dried figs 20 prunes 20 dried apricots

Source: Colgan Institute, San Diego CA.

your body, it burns a lot of fat.

Resistance exercise yields a further fat-loss bonus. It not only maintains muscle mass, it increases muscle, thereby providing more muscle cells in which fat will be burned.[23] It's a real health bargain. *Step 14: Do high-repetition, wide-variety resistance exercise.*

Exercise Intensity

In many, many gyms I see women especially doing high repetitions with weights so low they spend the whole workout chatting while exercising. That's pretend exercising. It does nothing at all.

The basic rules of muscle work are simple. If you use heavy resistance, so that you can complete only 3-6 repetitions of an exercise, and you do 5-6 sets, you build maximum strength but you don't lose much fat. If you set the weight so that you can just complete 8-12 repetitions, and you do 3-4 sets, you build muscle well and burn medium amounts of fat. If you set the weight so you run out of steam in 20-25 repetitons, and you do only one set, you build a little muscle and burn a lot of fat.

Step 15: for maximum fat-loss do one set of each exercise with a weight that exhausts you in 20-25 repetitions.

Timing Is Everything

You also need to know the right time to exercise. Despite all those calorie charts showing that running burns more calories than walking, and cross-country skiing burns most calories of all, fat loss has little to do with calories used during the exercise session. Numerous recent studies show that the right exercise raises your metabolic rate not only while you are doing it, but for up to 18 hours afterwards.[24,25]

If you exercise in the evenings and then go to bed, you lose most of the fat-loss effect, because sleep causes your metabolic rate to drop like a stone. So you have to exercise in the mornings, and the earlier the better.

Step 16: Exercise in the mornings.

Exercise Frequency

The number of exercise sessions per week is also crucial. Dr. Leonard Epstein analysed all the published studies on exercise and fat loss, and showed that folk who exercise five times weekly lose three times as much fat as those who exercise only twice or three times weekly, even if they exercise for longer. Those who exercised only once per week lost no fat at all.[26]

We have found the same result at the Colgan Institute. For fat loss, five days weekly of 30 minutes is much superior to three days weekly of 70 minutes, even though the total weekly exercise time of the three-day people is an hour longer. In order to keep that metabolic rate churning, frequent exercise is the key.

Step 17: Exercise five mornings weekly for a minimum of 30 minutes.

Antioxidants Stop Exercise Damage

As we saw in Chapter 14, oxidation is the primary mechanism of human degeneration. Because exercise uses 12-20 times more oxygen than sitting in a chair, it also creates masses of free radicals that do a lot of oxidation damage. Without additional antioxidants you are slowly killing yourself.

In order to reap the resistance exercise benefits of greater muscle and lower bodyfat, you have to combat exercise oxidation damage with antioxidant supplements. An average healthy person exercising for slimness and health (but not a competitive athlete), can overcome the extra oxidation caused by 5x30 minutes exercise per week, by taking a multiple antioxidant supplement. The Colgan Institute uses a supplement consiting of:

Beta-carotene	10,000 I.U.
Vitamin E (tocopherol complex)	200 I.U.
Vitamin E (d-alpha tocopheryl)	600 I.U.
Vitamin C (ascorbic acid)	1000 mg
Vitamin C (calcium ascorbate)	240 mg
Vitamin C (magnesium ascorbate)	200 mg
Vitamin C (ascorbyl palmitate)	200 mg
Zinc (picolinate)	15 mg
Selenium (selenomethionine)	200 mcg
Selenium (sodium selenite)	100 mcg
L-glutathione	50 mg
Coenzyme Q10	30 mg
Vegetable antioxidant complex	500mg

Step 18: Take a multiple antioxidant every day.

Special Fat Loss Supplements

The only compounds for weight loss approved by the FDA are **benzocaine** which reduces taste responses to food, and **phenylpropanolamine (PPA)** which suppresses appetite. But even the makers of these remedies don't recommend them for long-term weight control.

Don't despair. There's still a lot you can do without resorting to unhealthy prescription drugs or having your mouth wired up or your stomach stapled. Let's review some strategies that track human physiology from mouth to fat cells.

The first strategy is to reduce appetite. Phenylpropanolamine does that a bit. Better is **ephedrine hydrochloride** and its original herbal source *Ma huang or Ephedra sinica*. But use of these compounds should be very judicious. Any more than 25-50 mg per day of the active drug will cause quick habituation and loss of effect, and a host of side-effects including raised blood pressure, anxiety, and insomnia.

The second strategy is to reduce the taste of food, especially sweet tastes, so that you don't eat just for taste satisfaction. The herb *Gymnema silvestre* has been used for this purpose for thousands of years in Ayurvedic medicine. It works a bit.

The third strategy is to reduce your body's tendency to store fat. Another herb *Garcinia cambogia*, a specific variant of the English brindleberry, is used in Ayurvedic medicine for this purpose. The active ingredient is **hydroxy citrate**. Ongoing studies by Dr. Andrew Weil at the University of Arizona indicate that 500 mg of garcinia may reduce fat storage from a high-fat meal by up to 30%. Bonus: it may also reduce appetite.

The final strategy is to raise metabolic rate so that your body burns more calories all day long. This strategy is popularly called **thermogenesis**, which is just a fancy name for raising body temperature. To maintain the increased temperature, the body has to burn more calories to make the heat - lots of calories. And because it is low level activation, the calories burned come mainly from fat.[28]

Sounds ideal and there are tons of drugs that do the trick. But all of them have unhealthy side effects.[27] It is useless to lose fat if you make yourself unhealthy in the process.

Least damaging are the **beta-adrenergic agonists** and most innocuous of these is ephedrine or its herbal source *Ma huang*. These compounds work by increasing bodily output of noradrenalin, one of our fight-or-flight hormones. That should warn you right away not to use too much, (25-50 mg per day is plenty), or you run into severe anxiety, irritability, headache, and insomnia. The FDA are against ephedrine because some folk have used larger doses and caused real damage to the thyroid gland and other organs.

But ephedrine by itself is not effective anyway, because your body quickly defends itself with multiple mechanisms that turn off the extra noradrenalin. The three main defenses your body uses against a sensible ephedrine regimen (25-50 mg/day) are, increasing output of a chemical called adenosine, increasing output of phosphodiesterase enzymes, and increasing prostaglandin production.[14]

These defenses can be overcome respectively by using **caffeine, theophylline** (from tea) and **acetylsalicylic acid** (aspirin). Herbal sources can also supply the caffeine, theophyline, and aspirin. Standardized extracts of kola nut, guarana, black tea, and white willow are good sources.

And you can prolong the effect of caffeine, which incidentally is mildly thermogenic itself, by use of **naringenin** a compound found in grapefruit.[14]

Another effective chemical to use in conjunction with beta-receptor agonists is **yohimbine**, a compound from the bark of the yohimbe tree. Yohimbine is one of a class of compounds called **selective antagonists of alpha-2 receptors**. This action of yohimbine has been shown to cause long-term thermogenesis and fat-loss in animals.[14]

The last thing you can do to lose bodyfat is control excess

body water. Women especially have this problem. Bloating and edema inhibit your Lean For Life program because they make you feel blah, and induce you to sit like a slug and avoid exercise.

Diuretic drugs are not the solution, but mildly diuretic foods like melons, cucumber, grapes, apples, parsley, pineapple and cooked asparagus all help you shed excess water. Mild diuretic herbs such as Uva ursi and Sarsaparilla also have a use in this phase of fat-loss.
Step 19: Use the right herbal fat-loss supplement every day.

Goals Are The Key

Success never occurs in a vacuum. It is always tied to goals. To improve their performance, I get all athletes to set specific goals and sub-goals and write them down and post them for all to see.

Goals have to be specific, measurable, and time limited. "To lose weight" is hopelessly vague. "To lose 10 lbs of fat by my birthday," is the sort of goal you need.

Lean For Life is a very long-term goal, so sub-goals are essential to tell you how you are doing. If your birthday is four months away, then you have to lose a measured 2½ lbs each month, which is about the maximum you can achieve if you want to keep the fat off. Some athletes on our programs have a five-year goal of bodily improvement. To get there we set up to six sub-goals per year.

Finally, goals have to be public. Secret goals don't work. You have to be shamed and blamed for failure, and praised and rewarded for success. So make your goals public, and tie them to strongly desired rewards that are given only for success.
Step 20: Form specific, measurable, public, rewarded fat-loss goals.

Twenty Steps to Lean For Life

This has been a long chapter even to skim the effective strategies for fat-loss. But excess fat is your biggest health risk. So it's worth knowing every word. Table 12 presents a summary of the fat loss program used by the Colgan Institue. Our clients stick laminated copies on their refrigerators. Over 20 years we have led thousands of folk to grow lean for life, many who thought they were hopeless cases. If they can do it so can you. It's your passport to health and vitality.

> Half measures are 50% failure
> before they start.

Table 12: Twenty Steps To Lean For Life.

1. Lose no more than half-a-pound of fat per week.

2. Measure your bodyfat once a month.

3. Eat a low, low-fat diet.

4. Do not eat foods containing more than 20% fat calories.

5. Trust only the **Nutrition Facts** panel on foods.

6. Cut the sugar, eat complex carbohydrates instead.

7. Don't skip meals. Eat five small meals per day.

8. Avoid all fad diets.

9. Take a high quality multi-vitamin and multi-mineral every day.

10. Use a chromium picolinate supplement every day.

11. Use an l-carnitine supplement every day.

12. Eat 40 grams of mixed fibers every day.

13. Take a flax oil essential fatty acid supplement every day.

14. Do high repetition, wide variety resistance exercise.

15. Do one set of each exercise with a weight that exhausts you in 20-25 repetitions.

16. Exercise in the mornings.

17. Exercise five mornings weekly for a minimum of thirty minutes.

18. Take a multiple antioxidant every day.

19. Use the right herbal fat-loss supplement.

20. Form specific, measurable, public, rewarded fat-loss goals.

Chapter 25

Exercise: Essential Prevention

When not sleeping your body was designed to be almost continually active. Immobilize a limb for just three hours and it starts to degenerate. That's why even during sleep you automatically flex and stretch and turn more than a hundred times a night. *Disuse is deadly.*

How do we know? In 1982 Dr. Walter Bortz from the Department of Medicine at Palo Alto Medical Clinic, California, published an all important paper in the **Journal of the American Medical Association**. He reviewed over 100 studies showing that the sedentary lifestyle developed in the last 50 years in America causes widespread bodily damage.[1] This damage occurs independently of other health risk factors, such as smoking, alcohol, fat, age, and family history of disease.

Let's look at a few of his findings. By itself, simple inactivity causes a chain reaction of cardiovascular decay. First, it reduces *vital capacity*. That is, sitting like a slug reduces your ability to take up and use oxygen. So muscles, organs, and brain become partially oxygen deprived. Second, inactivity reduces cardiac output, that is, the ability of your heart to pump blood around the body. So the tissues of couch potatoes become doubly deprived. They get less oxygen and they get less blood and the essential nutrients blood contains.

In an effort to make up these deficits, your body constricts arteries, thereby raising blood pressure. This arterial constriction on top of a weakened heart not only increases the risk of clots and stroke, but also makes your cardiovascular system less able to respond to sudden movement or changes of position. Consequently, sedentary folk often suffer dizziness on standing, because the impaired system cannot instantly increase blood flow to the brain. With any sudden movements they are prone to falls and accidents, because the restricted system of blood flow cannot respond efficiently.

One of the most interesting studies shows that more sedentary people than active people are hit and killed in traffic accidents. No, it's not because a gang of crazed motorists hunts them down. It's because their weakened cardiovascular systems make them incapable of performing the nimble moves required to avoid oncoming traffic, without becoming dizzy and staggering or falling in the process. So when someone tells you that couch potatoes run mega-risks of being creamed by a truck - you better believe it.

Inactivity also increases levels of cholesterol and triglycerides. Triglycerides are the fats you store, and we have already seen in Chapter 24 how inactivity makes you fat.

In a vicious cycle, inactive muscles shrink to Pee Wee Herman size, compromising your ability to burn fat, to perform even simple tasks like running up stairs, and even to hold up your skeleton.

Bones also thin and weaken because your skeleton requires continuous resistance exercise in order to grow new bone matrix. As we saw in Chapter 13, a combination of inactivity and poor bone nutrition is the major cause of the epidemic of osteoporosis now burdening America - another man-made and entirely preventable disease.

Inactivity also disrupts bowel function and disorders glucose metabolism, independently of whatever food you eat. The near epidemics of intestinal disorders and adult-onset diabetes in America bear mute testimony to our slug lifestyle.

Sex hormone levels also decline with inactivity, now linked to the huge increase in impotence in America. As I show in my book **Sexual Potency**, the evidence is overwhelming that the incidence of male impotence in America has doubled since the 1940's.[2]

Exercise Can Save Your Life

I could go on listing the decay caused by disuse for many pages, but I think the examples given are enough. Bortz's work was a wake-up call to the medical community, that simply lounging about is one of the biggest risks to the nation's health. After his work appeared, the Norman Rockwell image of the chubby, rosy-cheeked physician disappeared from TV like smoke.

Since then, hundreds of new studies have presented dramatic evidence supporting Bortz. One of the best was conducted by renowned exercise guru Dr. Kenneth Cooper and colleagues, at his Aerobics Center in Dallas. They followed 13,344 men and women for fifteen years. This meticulous research, controlled for all major interfering variables such as age, family history, personal health history, smoking, blood pressure, cardiovascular condition, and insulin metabolism.

At the fifteen-year follow-up, reduced risk of death was closely correlated with physical fitness. This included deaths from cardiovascular diseases, a variety of cancers, and even accidents.[3] There is no longer any doubt: exercise can save your life, while couch potatoism creates an existence that is nasty, sick, and short.

Many folk still find it hard to accept that exercise directly prevents disease. So I will cover a few highlights of the evidence to convince the doubters.

Exercise Strengthens Heart and Lungs

Numerous studies show that exercise protects your body by maintaining vital capacity, and therefore maintaining adequate oxygenation of tissues.[4] The average sedentary American male aged 45 has lost half his ability to take up and use oxygen. With one year of the right exercise, he can restore it to the level of a 25 year old. Dr. Bortz rightly concludes that *the health benefits of restoring vital capacity are superior to any drug or medical treatment in existence.*[1]

In contrast to the weak cardiac function of sedentary folk, the athlete's strong, slow pulse is telling evidence of a healthy heart. Very few of the thousands of athletes and regular exercisers who have passed through the Colgan Institute in the last 20 years, have resting heart rates above 65 beats per minute. Many have rates in the 40s, and we once recorded champion cyclist Howard Doerfling at an incredible 29 beats per minute.

Sedentary folk, however, are likely to show heart rates in the 80s or 90s. As you can see from Figure 4, when heart rate rises above

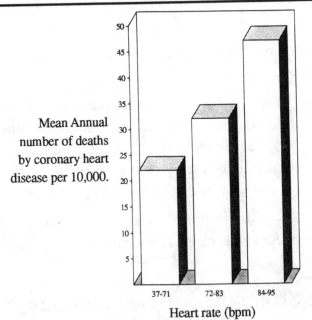

Mean Annual
number of deaths
by coronary heart
disease per 10,000.

Heart rate (bpm)

Figure 4. Resting heart rate and death by coronary heart disease. Adapted from Greenburg H, ed. **Sudden Coronary Death**. New York: NY Academy of Sciences, 1982;3-21.).

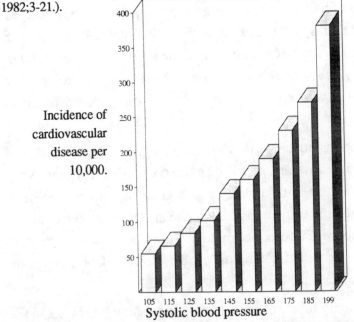

Incidence of
cardiovascular
disease per
10,000.

Systolic blood pressure

Figure 5. Systolic blood pressure and cardiovascular disease. Adapted from Laragh JH, et al, eds. **Frontiers in Hypertension Research**. New York, NY: Springer Verlag, 1981;17.)

84, risk of coronary heart disease more than doubles.

Exercise Protects Blood Pressure

What we used to regard as normal blood pressure, 120/80 mmHg, is not normal at all, only usual. That is, the majority of average folk show blood pressures of 120/80 mmHg. We know now that these people are already on their way to disease.

As Figure 5 shows, risk of cardiovascular disease starts to rise as systolic blood pressure goes above 103 mmHg. By 120 mmHg, previously thought to be normal, risk has risen from 51 to 77 per 10,000 people. That is an increase of 50%. By 135 mmHg, a level that many physicians still regard as marginal but acceptable, risk has doubled. Beyond 135 mmHg you are a walking time bomb.[5]

The same applies to diastolic blood pressure. Usual levels found in average folk are 80-89 mmHg. Recent research shows that these figures indicate a pre-disease state. Diastolic pressures below 80 mmHg, show an incidence of new cardiovascular disease of 10 cases per 1000. But diastolic pressures of 80-89 mmHg show an incidence of 40 cases per 1000, a 300% increase in risk of disease.[5]

Don't fret. It's easy to reduce blood pressure with the right exercise. At the Colgan Institute, 80% of subjects on our programs for one year or more, have resting blood pressures below 120/80 mmHg.

Numerous studies show that exercise works for older people too, in whom you might think the damage to blood pressure is permanent. In a typical study, Dr. A. Barry and colleagues followed sedentary hypertension patients aged 55 to 78 years.[5a] All had elevated blood pressure. After participating in an exercise program, systolic blood pressure fell by a whopping 20 mmHg. Regular exercise will lower blood pressure in almost anyone.

Exercise Lowers Cholesterol

Despite media bleatings, cholesterol is not the bad guy. Cholesterol is essential to every function of your body. It forms part of all your organs, including your heart and your brain. Your body makes all your steroid hormones, including adrenalin, estrogen and testosterone from cholesterol. You cannot live without it.

Most of your cholesterol is not from food at all. It is manufactured in your body mainly by your liver, every day of your life. When a *healthy* body eats high cholesterol foods, the liver immediately reduces its own cholesterol production to keep blood cholesterol low and healthy.[6]

It is disordered cholesterol metabolism that causes blood cholesterol to rise to dangerous levels. Disordered cholesterol metabolism is a man-made disease in America, caused predominantly by our degraded nutrition and sedentary lifestyle. I could spend pages discussing the "bad" low-density lipoprotein (LDL) cholesterol and the "good" high-density lipoprotein (HDL) cholesterol. But total cholesterol is mostly LDL and smaller particles, and this simple measure is still one of the best predictors of cardiovascular disease.[7] Total cholesterol has the added convenience that you can now measure it reasonably accurately at home with a simple device called the "Accumeter" for only $15.00.

But what level is healthy? In the mid '80s, the American Heart Association and other US health authorities made "below 200 mg/dl" their official recommendation. Today we know that even 200 mg/dl is too high. In the most comprehensive study yet, Dr. Jeremiah Stamler and colleagues followed 356,000 men in 28 US cities. As

Figure 6 shows, death rates from cardiovascular disease start to rise as cholesterol goes above 168 mg/dl.[8]

How do our sedentary citizens stack up? As Figure 7 shows, total cholesterol in average American men and women rise over 200 mg/dl in their 30s and reach about 220 mg/dl by age 45.[9] It's clear that sitting like a slug renders you ripe for disease.

How do athletes stack up? Recent research shows that average cholesterol levels in male and female bodybuilders and runners ranged between 158 mg/dl and 183 mg/dl.[10] Exercise sure makes the healthy difference.

I have spent a while showing how exercise protects you from cardiovascular diseases for two reasons. First, they are far and away our biggest disease problem, killing more than twice as many Americans as all cancers, nine times as many as all other lung and liver diseases combined, and 28 times as many as all forms of diabetes.[11] Alzheimers, osteoporosis, kidney diseases, multiple sclerosis, and other high profile disorders are all minor (except to the folk suffering them), and AIDS, despite all it's publicity, isn't even in the hunt.

The second reason for stressing cardiovascular protection by exercise is recent media distortions of the deaths of ill-informed folk who jump from long-term sedentary lifestyles into strenuous exercise programs. There are very good reasons for warning everyone contemplating exercise to get a thorough medical and physician's approval before they begin. As the **Johns Hopkins Medical Letter** says, sudden exertion in sedentary people "raises your chances of a heart attack . . . . 100-fold".[12] **The Mayo Clinic Health Letter** agrees, "Most people who have heart attacks during activity are sedentary or have underlying heart disease and overdo it".

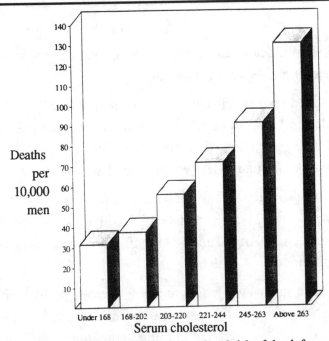

Figure 6. Correlation between serum cholesterol and risk of death from coronary heart disease in the next six years. (Stamler J, et al. **J Amer Med Assoc** 1986;256:2823-2828.)

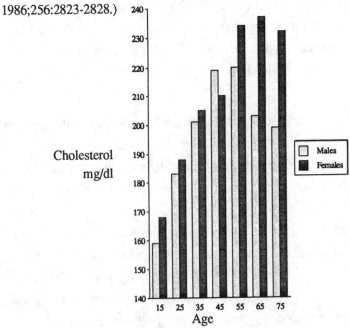

Figure 7. Average changes with age of serum cholesterol of Americans. (Derived from **The Metpath Reference Manual**. Teterboro, NJ: Metpath Inc, 1993.)

But if you do the right exercise four or five times per week for 30 minutes or more, then sudden exertion hardly increases your risk at all. So ignore media headlines that yet another jogger has dropped dead during training. It was likely his first exercise program for years.

Exercise Prevents Cancer

Most cancers are slow-slow-growing diseases, eating away silently at your body for years before they show themselves. Despite the overblown claims of successful treatment by the National Cancer Institute, once a cancer emerges medicine is usually powerless.

Any time you feel reassured by pronouncements of the cancer industry, remember the swift deaths of Michael Landon of pancreatic cancer, and Jaqueline Kennedy Onassis of lymphoma. If there was an effective treatment anywhere in the world, don't you think such immensely rich people would have bought it? So, if a little of the right exercise can prevent cancer, it's worth more than all the gold in Fort Knox. And like all the other best things in life - it's free!

I referred earlier to the study by Dr. Kenneth Cooper of 13,344 men and women followed for fifteen years.[3] After eliminating interfering factors, incidence of all forms of cancer was closely correlated with lack of physical fitness. Unfit men and women were 300% more likely to develop cancer. And the fitter that subjects were, over five levels of fitness, the lower their risk of cancer.

But the best finding from this study, is that you have to move only a smidgen out of couch potatoland to prevent cancer big time. As Dr. Carl Casperson of the Centers For Disease Control in Atlanta puts it, "You don't have to be a marathoner. A half-hour of exercise several days a week can drop your risk dramatically".[14]

I haven't space to cover the burgeoning pile of new studies showing that exercise inhibits specific cancers. So I will confine discussion to two pertinent examples, one solely for women and one mainly for men.

Breast cancer is the most frequent female cancer, and the third biggest cancer killer in America. And, as we saw in chapter 11, proportionately more women are developing and dying of breast cancer today than in the 1960s. Just to load the dice, we will add uterine cancer, ovarian cancer, and all other cancers of the female reproductive system. That's four of the leading six categories of female cancer. Together they wipe out 220,000 American women every year.[15] If simple exercise can help prevent such devastation, then it's a winner for every woman in the nation.

In a major study, Dr. Rose Frisch and colleagues at the Harvard School of Public Health, followed 5000 women college alumnae. Those who did regular, moderate exercise from high school on, had many fewer breast cancers and reproductive system cancers than their sedentary class mates.[16] This evidence is clear. Regular exercise can stop female cancers cold.

The major mechanism by which exercise prevents these cancers is regulation of estrogen and other sex hormones, which, left unchecked, cause uncontrolled cell proliferation in the female reproductive system.[15,16] It's likely that women who exercise regularly are simply activating an essential health mechanism in their bodies, designed to be activated in just that way by the miraculous hand that crafted all life upon the Earth.

What about exercise and male cancer? The examples I want to use are colon and rectal cancers, although these are also a leading cause of cancer death in women. Colo-rectal cancers are the second leading cancer category, with more than 155,000 new cases every year.[15] And incidence of these cancers has jumped since 1970. Red meats and animal fats are major causes, but so is inactivity.[17]

A huge study measured the exercise levels and the resting heart rates of 8000 men over 21 years. As we have seen, resting heart rate is a good measure of fitness and provides a good check on reported exercise. The risk of colon and rectal cancers was directly correlated with heart rate.[18]

An even larger study tracked 17,000 Harvard alumnae for 25 years. Subjects who were highly active, burning 2500 calories or more in exercise each week, showed only half the risk of colon cancer as their sedentary peers.[19]

The mechanism by which exercise probably prevents colorectal cancers is simple, and is also part of the human design. Exercise naturally promotes regular bowel movements, and increases the speed of excretion of food wastes. It therefore reduces time for carcinogen formation, and also prevents prolonged contact between carcinogens and intestinal walls. In our constipated society that spends a sickening $700 million a year on harmful (oops, "gentle, safe and soothing") laxatives, this sort of evidence should be a clarion call to exercise.[20]

These studies are just a fraction of the mass of meticulous research in respected medical journals showing that exercise prevents cancer. Yet I have in front of me a pile of public advice pamphlets from the National Cancer Institute and the American Cancer Society stretching back over the last decade. Nowhere in any of them is exercise even mentioned as protective against cancer. Of course, unlike pharmaceuticals and medical treatment, exercise is free and available to everyone. So it garners no grants, solicits no ads, and makes no obscene profits.

In the medical journal **CA** for example, the American Cancer Society's professional journal for physicians, a new analysis of risk factors for breast cancer includes everything from residence in northern states to socioeconomic class --- except couch potatoism.[21] I'll bet my new hiking boots against a spit in the wind, that inactivity causes far more breast cancers than living in North Dakota.

Anyone less trusting than I, might suspect that the geniuses who populate our health agencies, are either far too brilliant to bother with lowly scientific research, or they dance to more moving music. "One-step, two-step, I'll scratch you-step, If you'll scratch me-step, Tee Hee Hee-step."

Exercise Against All Disease

Only recently have medical scientists come to appreciate that the health benefits of exercise extend over a wide range of disorders. No! I'll stop pussyfooting and go right out on a limb. *The right exercise is a major strategy for preventing and treating ALL disease.* Physicians who do not incorporate exercise into their treatment protocols are guilty of malpractice.

I better back that up with strong evidence before some of my sedentary, disbelieving medical acquaintances have me drawn and quartered. I am thinking especially of three senior medical faculty members at Dalhousie University, who have allowed themselves to become so fat, that their love handles flop over and muffle their pagers. I'm not making it up. The love handle muffle was reported in the **New England Journal of Medicine**.[22]

We have discussed the evidence already that the right exercise maintains your heart, your lungs, your muscles, your bones, a healthy level of bodyfat, even your intestinal function. But what about more subtle functions, such as insulin, and your body's handling of sugar.

We have known for fifty years that couch potatoism leads to glucose intolerance.[23] Only recently, however, has research shown that getting off the couch, not only maintains insulin function to deal with the sugar, but also can reverse decades of damage. In insulin dependent diabetics for example, the right exercise programs increase insulin efficiency so much that some patients who have used daily insulin for years no longer need it.[24]

In healthy folk, the right exercise completely protects glucose tolerance against the degenerative changes in insulin metabolism that lead to adult-onset diabetes.[25] Old but healthy men who maintain a lifelong exercise program, have the same healthy insulin efficiency as young men.[26] The high-sugar American diet, which progressively destroys insulin metabolism, makes it virtually mandatory to exercise if you want to avoid glucose intolerance as you age.

What about age changes as subtle as hardening of the arteries, a degenerative process still believed by most physicians to be inevitable? At the National Institute on Aging Research Center in Baltimore, Maryland, Dr. Edward Lakatta and colleagues are showing in ongoing experiments, that regular exercise maintains arterial elasticity and even *reverses* arterial hardening that has already occurred.

I could go on for many pages citing one bodily function after another that is maintained by regular exercise. But I will cut to the chase. Recent research has revealed the major way in which exercise protects you against *all* disease. It started with evidence that exercise increases overall white cell counts in the blood.[27] Then came more precise findings, that moderate exercise increases bodily production of **lymphocytes, interleukin 2, neutrophils,** and other disease fighting components of the immune system.[27] There's no longer any doubt that the right exercise strengthens your immunity.

Hence it strengthens your resistance to all forms of damage, decay, bacteria, viruses, toxins, even radiation. Remember, the wise words of Louis Pasteur, the father of modern medicine, "Host resistance is the key".

The Right Exercise

All along I have stressed the *right exercise* because programs I see in gyms and health clubs across the nation are mostly wrong! wrong! wrong! It has also become eminently fashionable, and morally acceptable, for hordes of our citizens to emerge at dawn, clad in multi-colored underwear, complete with high-fashion fanny pack and fifty-function wristwatch, to join their identically clad neighbors in a stolid, trotting trudge against disease. For most of them, breathing the increased amounts of polluted air and subjecting their nutrient deprived bodies to the stress of running, does far more harm to their health than good.

In the mid-eighties, a vital clue to the right exercise for lifelong health was uncovered by brilliant research in an unexpected discipline - biochemistry. Biochemists established that all cell replication in the immune system, and therefore all immune strength, is dependent on availability of the amino acid **glutamine**.[28] Your immune system uses a ton of it.

But immune cells cannot make glutamine. Only muscle cells can do the job. So your muscles have to supply large amounts of glutamine to your immune system every day in order to maintain it.[29,30]

That's it. We have learned already that the mitochondria of muscle are the furnaces in which most of your bodyfat and sugar are burned for fuel. We have learned already that muscle is what stresses your skeleton to maintain your bones. Now we know that muscle is the vital link which also maintains your immunity, and hence your resistance to all disease. Muscle is the health engine.

What Are We Doing?

With such overwhelming evidence that muscular exercise is essential to health, what are we doing about it? A big fat zero. Pompous politicians and health administrators, most of them sporting generous bay windows, established a National Health Objective for America, to have 60% of adults engage in regular, vigorous, physical exercise by 1990. When that failed to happen, the objective was blithely reset for the year 2000. It will never happen.

Such self-serving political poppycock would be comical if it were not so bad for the nation's health. If the National Health Objective on Exercise were serious, then there would be tremendous public incentives to drive it. There are none. As of today, fewer than 10% of American adults do any regular exercise at all.[31]

Our children are also being set up for sickly adult life. Despite Arnold Schwarzenegger's efforts with schools, the latest survey of grades 9-12 in all 50 states, shows that only one child in three meets the minimum standard of exercise: three times weekly for 20 minutes. That's a big *decline* since 1984 when 62% of children met the standard.[32] For health's sake, don't allow yourself or your children to be part of the couch potato brigade.

Muscle Is The Health Engine

Americans who *do* exercise mostly do aerobic forms such as walking, jogging, cycling, swimming, and aerobics classes. We have seen already that aerobic exercise provides insufficient resistance to maintain muscle. It's no wonder then that between the ages of 20 and 40 the average American woman loses 8 lbs of muscle and gains 23 lbs of fat. By 40 her immunity is seriously compromised.

Between ages 20 and 80 the average male loses a quarter of his total muscle mass. And his immunity goes down the tubes along with it.[33]

Weight-bearing exercise is the key. A pile of new studies show that it is vastly superior. Let's take some typical examples. Let's look at the cardiovascular system, because that is where aerobic exercise is supposed to shine.

Dr. Neil McCartney and colleagues at McMaster University, Ontario compared a ten-week program of weight training plus aerobic exercise, against aerobic exercise alone in patients with coronary heart disease. At the start of the study, the two groups of patients were similar in exercise capacity. The aerobic group did two sessions a week of 75 minutes of aerobic exercise. The weight training plus aerobic group did two sessions of 35 minutes weight training, then aerobics to bring their total exercise time to 75 minutes. So both groups spent exactly the same time exercising.

Results put aerobic exercise to shame. The aerobic group showed a negligible 2% increase in cardiovascular capacity, and only an 11% increase in endurance, measured as the time to exhaustion, on the stationary bike. The weight training group showed a 15% increase in cardiovascular capacity, and a massive 109% increase in endurance.

In strength, the results were even better for weight training. The aerobic group showed no strength increases in arm curl, leg press, and leg extension tests. The weight training group showed big increases: arm curl, 43%; leg press, 21%; and leg extension, 24%.[34]

What about fat loss. The ocean of fat booties I see bobbing up and down three inches on stair-steppers, and oscillating in aerobics classes, indicate that most women still believe in aerobics for moving the flab. But we have to bow to the evidence. A typical study compared the bodyfat of sedentary women against women who exercise aerobically and women who do resistance exercise.[35] Results showed:

- Sedentary women - 21.8% bodyfat.

- Aerobic exercisers - 16.2% bodyfat.

- Resistance exercisers - 14.7% bodyfat. 'Nuff said.

We have already seen in Chapter 13 that aerobic exercise also fails to maintain your bones, and that weight-bearing exercise does the job easily. And most important of all, aerobics cannot maintain muscle. Weight training not only maintains but also increases muscle mass, thereby providing a more plentiful supply of glutamine for your immunity. You have to move some weights if you want a long and healthy life.

We can't claim to be the only researchers who have come to this realization, although the Colgan Institute has advocated weight-bearing exercise for health since 1982, so we were one of the first. The American College of Sports Medicine didn't change its advice on aerobic exercise until the '90s. Now, Dr. Worthy of their Advisory Board states:

"Done correctly weight training is the most efficient, effective, and safest form of exercise there is, and it won't be long before people realize it."[36]

I hope the evidence has convinced you.

How To Exercise

First, get a clearance from your physician. Never begin an exercise program without it. Then, *start easy*. Don't jump into a vigorous weight program which involves health clubs and special periods out of your working day. It has a 95% risk of failure. It takes too much of your time. It becomes an added life burden.

And it's no good loading all your exercise into one day a week. It doesn't work. To be successful, exercise must be incorporated into your normal daily routine. Fifteen minutes a day when you rise in the mornings, is far better for your health than three hours at a gym on Saturdays.

You don't need complicated machines or fancy gadgets. You can exercise anywhere. Your own body weight and gravity provide ample resistance. Gradual, progressive exercise is best. There is no need to steam, no need to work to your limit.

Never strain. Anytime you ache next day, you are going too hard. *The body does not need to be inflamed in order to improve*. Inflammation is counter-productive. Overtraining is de-training.

Remember, you are limited by the rhythms of Nature. Adaptation is slow - but sweetly sure. The first day you begin exercising, even after doing none for thirty years, your body starts to rejuvenate.

Your exercise program has three goals. First and most important is to maintain and increase your muscle mass. Second is to maintain your cardiovascular system. Third is to maintain your flexibility. Mr. Average stiffens as he ages, increasing the risks of all sorts of strains and tendon, ligament and skeletal disorders.

Once you have your physician's clearance to exercise, there is nothing wrong with a little aerobics, especially to warm-up the system and get your blood pumping. And twenty minutes at even mild intensity will have cardiovascular benefits. We advocate aerobics to begin exercise for everyone, because you should never pick up weights cold. Then 5-10 minutes spent stretching after your muscles are warm, is all you need to maintain flexibility lifelong.

Now you are ready for muscle. Your program should include resistance exercise for shoulders, arms, chest, back, legs and abdominals. If you are doing three days per week, which is the starting level and the minimum for consistent benefit, then do:

Day 1 - Shoulders and Arms

Day 2 - Chest and Back

Day 3 - Legs and Abdominals

If you are doing five days per week, the optimum program for health, then do one bodypart per day:

Day 1 - Shoulders

Day 2 - Arms

Day 3 - Chest

Day 4 - Back

Day 5 - Legs and Abdominals

Some secrets that will give you faster progress and a better body than most people you see in health clubs.

1. No matter what the gym trainers say, Never do more per exercise than *one warm-up set* of 12 -15 easy repetitions, followed by *one medium heavy set* of 6-10 repetitions to exhaustion.

2. Work a bodypart only *once* per week. Exercised muscle takes about 48 hours to breakdown worn cells, then about 48-72 hours to build new, stronger replacements. That's five days. From 5-8 days strength remains at maximum and then slowly declines. So exercising a muscle very 5-8 days is the optimum program for progress.

3. Do not train with weights for more than *one hour* per workout. Your anabolic potential, that is, your ability to gain lean mass, is limited by your hormone levels. After 45 minutes to an hour, hormone levels decline. You may be able to will yourself to continue but it will not do your body any good.

4. Do as wide a *variety* of exercises as possible. Restricted resistance exercises, especially on machines, stress only certain fibers of a muscle in certain positions. You want to get all the fibers in all positions.

5. In one hour at two sets per exercise you can comfortably do *12 exercises*. Don't push to do more. Programs of the best exercises are available from the Colgan Institute at nominal cost. For those wishing to scan the whole range of possible weight exercise, I recommend my friend Bill Pearl's book, **The Encyclopedia on Weight Training**.[37]

6. Emphasize the *eccentric contraction* of each repetition. That is, the return phase of the repetition, when the muscle in question is lengthening under load. In a barbell bicep curl for example, the eccentric contraction occurs when you are lowering the bar to the

start position. Fight it all the way down, because it is the stress of lengthening under load that causes most of the strength and lean mass gains that you are seeking. When you see all those folk allowing weights to drop back to the start position, smile. You know better.

7. Increase your protein intake by taking a *protein drink* daily within one hour after workout. Much new research shows that weight training puts subjects into protein deficit, despite the high protein level of the American diet.[38]

8. Take daily antioxidant supplements. All exercise increases oxidation in the body.[38]

9. Eat an alkaline diet. All exercise increases body acidity. See the table of acid and alkaline foods in Chapter 13.

10. Sip a cold, light carbohydrate drink (7-10%) throughout workkouts. Drinks containing a little glucose, a little zylitol plus mostly glucose polymers are best. It will trickle carbohydrate continuously into your blood and spare your muscle glycogen, thereby maintaining your energy level. It will also prevent dehydration. As I show in my book **Optimum Sports Nutrition**, even 3% dehydration can reduce strength by 10%.[38] And it will help keep your body temperature down, thereby reducing the amount of blood diverted to the skin for cooling, thus leaving more to supply your muscles with oxygen and nutrients.

The final point to make about weight-bearing exercise is that without it, without the stimulus to your body to grow, nutritional supplements cannot work properly. Important new research just published in the **New England Journal of Medicine** shows that multi-vitamin and mineral supplementation had little effect in improving the health of old people. But when a resistance exercise program was added, the health benefits were astonishing, ranging from over 100% improvement in strength and muscle size to big improvements in mobility and recreational activity.[39]

It takes a bit of puff and stickability to grow a high-performance body. But once you've done it, the modicum of exercise necessary to maintain it is one of life's greatest bargains.

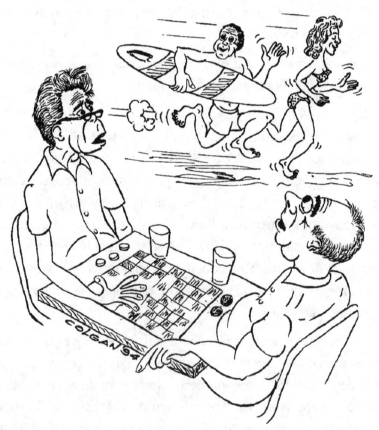

"Fred's no fun any more. Since he went on that antioxidant kick all he wants to do is play with my grandaughter."

Chapter 26

Save Your Brain

The most devastating disorder of all is to lose your mind. Most folk who become senile, develop Alzheimers, or other irreversible forms of brain degeneration *know* it is happening. Their anguish is far worse than physical pain. Progressive senility is living death, turning the most brilliant professors, the greatest athletes, the most gifted artists, into dribbling zombies. The worst of it is, we do most of the damage to ourselves.

The ten billion nerve cells of your brain process such uncountable amounts of information each second, they make our most advanced computers look like children's toys. Your brain controls everything, from the merest wiggle of toes, to the moment-to-moment balancing of hundreds of hormones, to the microscopically regulated metabolism of all the thirty trillion cells that enable you to think, feel, and behave as a human being. When even a few thousand brain cells get damaged or die, your whole body suffers.

As progressive brain damage accumulates, from poor

nutrition, bodily pollution, over-use of man-made drugs, and lack of exercise, intelligence declines, memories fade, muscles atrophy, bones weaken, immunity disappears, and you become aged and easy prey for every passing disease.

The ultimate solution to disease clearly lies in preventing degeneration of the brain. By the turn of this century much of medical science will be pointed in that direction. The good news is, that even now recent nutrition science has discovered significant ways to maintain and even improve brain function.

Nutrition Aids Memory

The first brain function to go is memory, beginning in Mr. Average about age 30 and accelerating after age 40.[1] You can change your behavior, improve your skills, enhance your life, only to the extent that you can store new information in long-term memory and recall it. If that capacity declines, you become an automaton, unable to learn anything new, forever re-enacting the habits and memories of an increasingly distant past.

To prevent this decline it is necessary to know a little about the structure of the nerves (**neurons**) in the brain. Each neuron consists of a stringy filament called a **dendrite**, then a cell body, then another stringy filament called an **axon** (see Figure 8). The dendrite carries nerve impulses towards the cell body, and the axon carries them away again. The nerve impulses carry the information, much like the electrical impulses that carry your spoken information along a phone line.

Unlike phone lines however, neurons are all unconnected to each other. The end of the axon of each neuron stops near the ends of dendrites of other neurons. The gap between the axon and

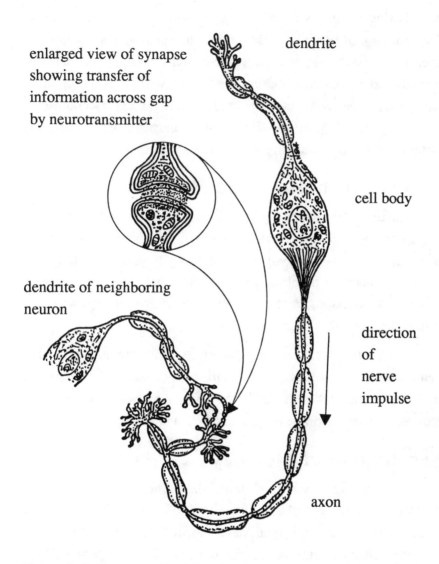

enlarged view of synapse showing transfer of information across gap by neurotransmitter

dendrite

cell body

dendrite of neighboring neuron

direction of nerve impulse

axon

Figure 8. Schematic of a brain neuron. Arrow shows direction of nerve impulses. Enlarged synapse view shows neurotransmitter particles released from the end bulb of the axon flowing to the neighboring dendrite of another neuron, thereby transmitting information across the synapse.

neighboring dendrites is called a **synapse,** as shown in Figure 8. Transmission of nerve impulses across the synapse is accomplished chemically by release of **neurotransmitters**, compounds that flow from the axon to the neighboring dendrites. Two of these compounds known to be involved in memory are **serotonin** and **acetylcholine**.[2,3] Both are formed from specific essential nutrients that your body cannot make. You must obtain them from your diet.

Neurotransmitters and Memory

Numerous studies show that learning is stored as memory largely through modification of synapses.[4,5,6] The particular pattern of synaptic discharges evoked by learning new information, sensitizes the neurons involved to trigger that pattern more easily on subsequent occasions. When the pattern recurs, memory of what was learned recurs also.

The important new finding is that the amount of a neurotransmitter present at the synapse, determines whether or not memory storage takes place. If the amount of neurotransmitter is reduced, memory storage is disrupted. We will look first at serotonin.

Serotonin and Memory

In an elegant series of animal experiments at the Center for Neurobiology at Columbia University, Professors Eric Kandel and James Schwartz and colleagues have shown that memory storage can be increased by putting additional serotonin into the neuron.[2,7] In humans also, we know that periods of additional serotonin release improve memory storage.

You can improve your memory, for example, if you sleep immediately after studying. This effect used to be explained by the common sense theory that sleeping cuts off all further input, and thus prevents interfering material from blocking storage of the learning. Now we know that the neurotransmitters are more important. Serotonin is released into the brain in large quantities as you fall asleep. It is probably the additional serotonin that improves the memory storage.

Drugs that increase brain serotonin also enhance memory. In one study, normal volunteers were fed alcohol on a number of occasions and then tested. All showed the usual alcohol-induced memory deficits. On other occasions, they were also given the drug **zimelidine**, which causes greater concentrations of serotonin at synapses. Result: no memory deficit from the alcohol.[8]

A mass of similar evidence shows clearly that increasing brain serotonin improves memory. Serotonin (5-hydroxytryptophan) is formed in brain neurons from the essential amino acid **l-tryptophan**, unfortunately now banned by the FDA. The rate of serotonin formation is controlled by the amount of l-tryptophan available to the brain from the blood.[9]

You can raise your blood tryptophan easily by eating tryptophan either in proteins or as a pure l-tryptophan supplement.[9] Folk in European countries have free access to this essential amino acid.

Because of the blood/brain barrier, however, only an l-tryptophan supplement will raise **brain** tryptophan without difficulty. Transport of amino acids across the blood/brain barrier is very limited. Tryptophan is one of the class of **large neutral amino acids (LNAAs)** that rely on a specific transporter molecule. If you eat protein food at the same time as l-tryptophan, then the other LNAAs in the food, **isoleucine, leucine, valine, tyrosine and phenylalanine** all compete with tryptophan for transport, so only a fraction gets through.[10] Alas, Americans have access to high amounts of l-tryptophan only in protein foods such as turkey.

You can get round this problem somewhat, by "neutralizing" the other LNAAs in the blood, by eating some high carbohydrate food at the same time as the protein, such as whole-grain bread, or rice cakes. Carbohydrate lowers blood levels of all the LNAAs, except tryptophan, thereby permitting it to enter the brain preferentially and so raise serotonin levels.[11] Your memory will surely benefit.

Acetylcholine and Memory

As memory declines with age, so does brain acetylcholine. This biochemical deficit is especially evident in the post-morten brains of people who had suffered the severe memory problems of premature senility or Alzheimers disease.[1] Biopsies from living patients also show greatly reduced capacity to make acetylcholine.[12] Aged people who have retained clear memory show much smaller deficits.[13]

Studies using drugs to block acetylcholine synthesis in the brain, provide further strong evidence that optimum acetylcholine levels are crucial to good memory. Young, normal subjects given the cholinergic blocker **scopolamine**, show memory deficits similar to Alzheimers patients, especially deficits in recent memory and in ability to learn new information.[14,15]

Working in the opposite direction, studies using drugs or nutrients to increase brain acetylcholine levels, have found substantial improvements in memory, not only in patients with memory loss, but also in normal subjects.[16] For example, after a single injection of the drug **arecholine**, which stimulates acetylcholine function, normal young adults showed greatly improved ability to learn and recall new material.[17]

Studies with nutrients have not been so successful. Brain acetylcholine is made from choline and pantothenic acid in the diet. The amount available to brain neurons is correlated with the amounts of these nutrients eaten, especially the choline.[18] However, numerous independent studies, feeding up to 20 grams of choline a day for up to two months to memory loss patients have found improvements in only a few subjects.[3]

Review of these studies by the Colgan Institute indicates five reasons why they may have failed. First, they did not use supplementary pantothenic acid, which is essential for acetylcholine formation. As we have seen throughout this book, increasing one nutrient drastically without increasing its co-factors cannot bring an optimum result.

Second, the diets of patients were not monitored or improved. As I have reported previously,[19] diets of elderly people are often deficient in numerous nutrients, including folic acid, vitamin B_{12} and thiamin. Any of these deficits can cause severe memory loss.[19] Any strategy to maintain or improve memory must be based on *complete nutrition*.

Third, post-mortems on memory loss patients usually show brain damage. The brain damage in the living patients treated with choline is unknown, but highly likely. It is useless to flood a brain with acetylcholine, if the neurons whose function it is supposed to improve are already dead.

Studies on patients and on normal subjects support this

inference. Dr. J.L. Signoret at Hôpital de la Salpetriere in Paris has shown that patients with *early* memory loss improve on choline, whereas patients who have shown memory loss for more than four years do not.[20] It seems likely that early memory loss patients still retain functional neurons on which the choline can act.

This explanation seems even more likely with the finding of Dr. N. Sitaram that ten grams of choline chloride can improve memories of normal, young adults.[17] These findings not only support the idea that choline supplementation must begin before the relevant brain cells die, but also suggest that if you want to maintain your memory, then begin early, before degeneration sets in.

The fourth reason why studies with choline mostly fail is lack of mental stimulation. In biochemical studies, increased choline in the diet reliably causes enhanced acetylcholine synthesis in the brain, *only if the relevant brain areas are stimulated*.[18] In all cases of successful choline enhancement of memory in normal men, the men were students who were studying, therefore getting intense mental stimulation. In the unsuccessful studies, with patients or average folk no attempt was made to stimulate brain function.

New evidence presented in **Science** in March 1994 indicates that, just as with every other part of the body, neurons require regular exercise in order to survive.[21] As with every other type of nutritional enhancement of function, nutrition alone is not sufficient. You sit like a slug, you grow to think like a slug. Exercising the brain appears to be a necessary condition for maintenance.

The final reason the choline studies mostly fail is they are not long enough. To expect to restore memory function in two weeks or even two months (the longest studies) seems ludicrous, when you consider that the brain deficit has taken twenty years or more to build up. You might get some minor improvements, but it is likely that major corrections require new growth of dendrites and axons, and even growth of whole new neurons.

Yes, I did mean new. This is heresy to many physicians who learned in medical school that you cannot grow new cells in the central nervous system. Well, science today has shown that you can.

Dr. Fernando Nottebohm and colleagues have made this remarkable discovery from animal studies. Animals given brain stimulating drugs and intense mental stimulation grow new brain cells and connections in adulthood.[22] Nottebohm believes it is likely that humans can do it too. This wonderful finding is completely contrary to the accepted dogma that brain cells do not regenerate, and what you got at birth is all you get. This new evidence suggests that anyone has a chance to improve the brain.

But it doesn't happen overnight. Extrapolating in cavalier fashion from Nottebohm's experiments and other studies, we estimate that human memory improvement, which requires new brain neurons and processes, may take a minimum of ten months and as much as six years of acetylcholine enhancement.

I am not saying that acetylcholine will directly cause new neuron growth. All I can say is that increased acetylcholine at the synapses, should yield more frequent, more efficient neural transmission, which in turn provides a stimulus for new growth.

In attempting to raise brain acetylcholine, you can't simply increase your intake of **lecithin** as is widely suggested in the health foods market. Store bought lecithins tested by the Colgan Institute contain very little choline. Dr. John Fernstrom, neurobiochemistry expert at MIT has similar findings.[11] Only **phosphatidyl choline** will work. We use the best available which is reliably 80% phosphatidyl choline. Supplements used in successful experimental studies range from 3-20 grams per day.

Antioxidants Maintain Your Brain

The next big discovery about the brain is that much of the damage to brain cells occurs by oxidation.[23] In addition to the antioxidants we have discussed previously, European research shows that the amino acid **acetyl-l-carnitine** maintains brain function partly by antioxidant action. Note, this is NOT l-carnitine but *acetyl*-l-carnitine.

More than 50 controlled studies show that this remarkable nutrient has profound effects in addition to antioxidant action. It improves memory, prevents brain cell loss, boosts intelligence, and restores acetylcholine metabolism. It is used in millions of doses of 1000-2000 mg per day throughout Europe, for treatment of Alzheimers, depression, and memory loss in the aged, and for improvement of cognition in normal folk.[24]

Acetyl-l-carnitine has recently become a popular nutrient at life extension clinics in the US. But of course, the FDA deny it has any effects at all. As this book goes to press you can still buy it over the counter here. Better stock up. As with all new and effective nutrients, it will soon be banned, until some pharmaceutical company can get a use patent or other frippery license to exploit its profit potential.

There are a dozen other nutrients based on amino acids, such as alpha-ketoglutaric acid, that have proven effects in maintaining your brain. But that is a whole other story which I will tell you in detail in my forthcoming book **Stop Aging**.

If you choose to organize your nutrition and exercise around this present book, **Stop Aging** is your next step. There are many recent and wonderful discoveries that can boost your brain power, your intelligence, your memory, and your health. Best of all, you will be able to apply these findings to your life in plenty of time to enjoy the breathtaking changes that will overtake Mother Earth by the turn of the new millennium.

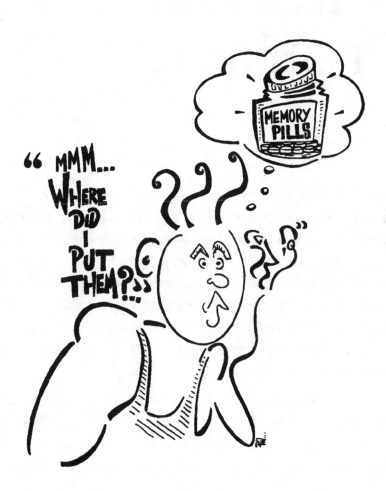

Chapter 27

Your Personal Nutrition Program

"**B**acteria ate my face", screamed recent headlines. No, its not some bogus tabloid tale. It's true. Mutations of the simple streptococcous A bacterium, responsible for endemic "strep throat" in America, have developed flesh-eating appetites that make Dracula look like a kindly uncle. They excrete an enzyme called **cystine protease** that can dissolve flesh. Faces might be fixable, but these virulent bugs will just as happily munch a lung, a kidney or a liver. In a recent outbreak in England, 70% of cases were resistant to all antibiotics and proved fatal.

The Centers for Disease Control in Atlanta have been monitoring this mutation in strep A since 1986. They estimate that the incidence in America has jumped to 15,000 cases per year, many misdiagnosed as everything from AIDS to radiation poisoning.[1] As usual, we did it to ourselves.

Antibiotic Misuse

You can't protect yourself with antibiotics. Misuse of these "wonder" drugs, which used to be very effective in their proper place of health crisis intervention, likely caused the Strep A mutations in the first place. Our out-of-control disease industry has created most of the new bugs that now plague us. Our physicians are unwittingly engaging in biological warfare against the American public, far worse than anything done by Saddam Hussein.

It happens by selective breeding. Each unnecessary prescription of an antiobiotic kills off the weak members of any bacterial colony that happens to be present (including the beneficial bacteria in your intestines). Only the strongest bacteria survive. With the competition for space and food removed, these resistant bugs multiply rapidly. Repeated misuse of different antiobiotics against a particular bacterial strain, quickly breeds bugs that are resistant to all of them.

Worse, wrongful use of antibiotics against self-limiting infections, hitting the flea with a sledgehammer, never allows your immune system to develop its own powerful resistance. Most children in America today have their immunity compromised by antibiotics wrongfully prescribed for every scratch and sniffle. It's a shameful indictment of medicine, to see multitudes of our offspring with ear drains and repeated ear, nose, and throat infections, against which they have never been allowed to develop resistance, because of massive use of unnecessary drugs.

Alexander Fleming, the discoverer of penicillin, told us many years ago of these potential problems. In 1981, when the crisis first loomed, a group of 150 scientists led by microbiologist Dr. Stuart Levy of Tufts University, warned that unless we apply antibiotics correctly, *"we may find a time when they are no longer useful to combat disease"*.[2]

Well, Dr. Levy, we didn't heed the warning, and the crisis is now upon us. In 1992 alone, physicians wrote over 4,000,000 useless antibiotic prescriptions for the common cold and 'flu viruses. They continue this malpractice year in year out, despite clear instructions in the **Physicians Desk Reference** that the drugs are effective only against *bacteria*.

That's nothing compared with hospitals. Recent studies show that up to *half* of all antibiotic use in American hospitals is improper.[4,5] This criminal malpractice, which I have seen myself in some of our best hospitals, has bred hundreds of man-made, antibiotic resistant bugs, including new strains of tuberculosis, pneumonia, E coli, salmonella, and meningitis.[5] They make hospitals very dangerous places to be.

Build Your Immunity

Bacteria provide just one graphic example, but the message is clear. As we have seen throughout this book, nutrients and exercise have many specific effects against specific diseases. But the most important effect is to strengthen immunity against *all* disease. Your first step in a personal health program is to build your immunity.

Think always, *"host resistance is the key"*. To strengthen yours, avoid any unnecessary use of medications, especially antibiotics, and any unnecessary contact with hospitals and medical facilities.

For the same reason avoid all but organically grown meats.

Antibiotics are massively misused in meat and poultry production. Eating them you get a double-whammy blow to your health, from the antibiotic residues in the meat, and from the antibiotic resistant bacteria it carries.

To help you further, I will tell you three strategies we use at the Colgan Institute to boost immunity. As with everything in this book, I can't advise you to use them. That is the exclusive function of your physician. But I can advise you to obtain the medical references and present them to your physician for appraisal.

In addition to a complete nutrition supplement and regular weight-bearing exercise, the first strategy is *P'au D'Arco* tea. This is a traditional South American herbal remedy made from the inner bark of the **purple lapacho**, an Argentinian tree. It is used there against a wide range of infections. In the 1960's a chemical called **naphthoquinone**, extracted from purple lapacho, was shown to have strong anti-viral, anti-bacterial and anti-fungal actions.[6]

We have used P'au D'arco for all types of acute infections, in place of antibiotics, for the last 15 years. Even babies can drink the tea mixed with fruit juice. There are no side-effects from P'au D'arco and it does not compromise immunity. Our children, and many thousands whose parents we have told about P'au D'arco, are raised antibiotic-free. *Caveat emptor.* There are numerous false P'au D'arcos sold on the herbal market. Only the Argentinian material is effective.

The second strategy is a simple amino acid. As we have discussed, strong immunity requires a lot of glutamine. An amino acid we use to boost the supply is **ornithine alpha-ketoglutarate** (OKG). Unlike l-glutamine itself, OKG is stable and does not raise body ammonia levels.

The third strategy is ion exchange whey protein concentrate. As we saw in Chapter 20, the protein in whey is a powerful immune booster. When you buy a protein drink look for one whose main ingredient is specifically whey protein concentrate.

Eat A Low Fat Diet

Low-fat intake is not only directly protective against cardiovascular disease and cancers, even skin cancer,[7] and in keeping down bodyfat, it also boosts immunity.[8]

Keep your fat intake to 15% of daily calories, preferably as organic olive oil or flax oil. Avoid all saturated and trans fats. Read the new nutrition panel on food labels.

Eat A Low Salt Diet

Sodium excess causes hypertension in sensitive individuals, increases the risk of stomach cancer,[9] and increases the risk of osteoporosis.[10]

Use a potassium based salt substitute on the table and in cooking. Keep your sodium below one gram a day.

Avoid Red Meats

Rates of colon cancer in America are ten times those of many Eastern nations. For 1990 new cases exceeded 150,000.[11]

In a massive clinical trial of 88,751 women, Dr. Walter Willett and colleagues at Harvard have shown that women who eat beef, pork, or lamb daily have a 250% increased risk of colon cancer.

Red meat consumption is now also linked to prostate cancer in a new study of 14,916 physicians.[13] Ditch the steak and chops. Your health will benefit.

Eat A High Fiber Diet

Fiber protects the colon from cancer, lowers cholesterol,[14] and stabilizes blood sugar.

Eat 40-50 grams of mixed fibers daily, as whole-grain breads and cereals, especially those containing oat bran, vegetables and fruits.

Eat A Low Sugar Diet

Refined sugars cause obesity, tooth decay, metabolic and cardiac abnormalities,and also increase the risk of adult-onset diabetes.[15]

Use a little fructose in place of table sugar. It is much sweeter than sucrose, so you use a lot less. Look for carbohydrate drinks sweetened with zylitol.

Eat Organic, Unprocessed Foods

We have stressed the degraded and contaminated nature of foods grown on NPK fertilizers, and foods processed for mass production. They do more harm than simply failing to provide nutrients. In order to use them, your body has to rob its own tissues of essential nutrients, to use in absorption and metabolism of any refined food.[15]

Avoid Processed Meats

Pickled, salt-cured, smoked, nitrated and charcoal-cooked meats contain potent carcinogens.[15] Don't eat them. At the barbecue don't allow the meats to char, and cut off any mistakenly charred bits.

Drink Clean Water

As we have seen, most American drinking water is now contaminated with any number of the 60,000 man-made chemicals that now pollute our ground water.

Drink bottled distilled or home-distilled water. Drink 8-10 glasses per day. Clean water is the best diluter of toxins there is.

Eat An Alkaline Diet

Acidity is an endemic disorder in America that causes much disease. Use the table in Chapter 13 to eat a more alkaline diet.

Limit Alcohol

Evidence shows clearly that a little alcohol is cardio-protective and also reduces effects of stress.[15] Drink no more than two glasses of wine *or* two beers *or* two singles of spirits per day.

Use The Pyramid

The Eating Right Pyramid should form the basis of your diet. Main foods for health are grains and cereals followed by vegetables, then fruits. Meats, eggs, fish, dairy products, and nuts should be treated as optional foods and kept to 15-20% of daily calories. Fats, oils and sweets should be used as garnish only.

Eat Variety

Each day new science uncovers new healthful compounds in foods. There are certainly many more we do not know of. Eating a wide variety of foods gives you the best chance of obtaining these nutrients. It also prevents the development of food sensitivities.

Take Daily Supplements

I hope the evidence has convinced you that nutrient supplements are essential for optimum health in these dog days of degraded and contaminated food and polluted water and air. It will get a lot worse before it gets better.

Protect yourself every day with a complete multi-vitamin, a complete multi-mineral, a potent multi-antioxidant and some essential fatty acids taken as organic flax oil.

Do Weight Bearing Exercise

Develop a lifelong program of weight-bearing exercise. And do it at least three times per week. Your heart, your lungs, your organs, your muscles, your bones, and your immunity cannot help but benefit.

Eliminate Toxic Metals

Until 1986 lead pipes were allowed for our water. Many of them still exist. It took fifty years to get the lead out of gasoline and water, and to convince government lead was damaging our children's brains. It will take another twenty years at least, to convince them about aluminum.

Aluminum causes multiple forms of brain damage and is now strongly linked with Alzheimers.[16,17] Eliminate it from your life in water, cooking, utensils, antacids and personal care items such as anti-perspirants and shampoos. For other toxic metals see my books **Prevent Cancer Now**,[11] and **Your Personal Vitamin Profile**.[15]

That's the whole health strategy until my book **Stop Aging** is published in 1995. But there's one more topic you need to know well. It's covered in the last chapter.

Chapter 28

Will The Truth Out?

Why don't we hear of most of the strategies in this book from our health authorities and large commercial companies? Simple. There's little money to be made from them. Kellog's, for example, makes plenty enough money from its Frosted Flakes, surely the most nourishing, disease-preventing food in existence, to spend $34 million annually just to promote it. In contrast, the National Cancer Institute spends only $400,000 annually to promote the potent cancer prevention effects of fruits and vegetables. No prime time TV ads here. Just dull little brochures crammed with spider writing.

For the same reason it makes no national headlines when the most eminent cardiovascular researcher in America, Dr. William Castelli, says,

> "I have not seen one case of coronary heart disease in anyone with a cholesterol count under 150."[1]

Only a good nutrition and exercise program can keep your cholesterol that low, and there's no specific medical profit to be made from that. Currently used medical diets and drugs to lower cholesterol are mostly a failure.[2,3]

But we will not be told these facts by health authorities. We have to realize that our lucrative health-care industry today, would go bankrupt if it was reduced to treating people in robust health who occasionally become ill. It is therefore highly motivated to maintain the American population in marginal health, prey to all kinds of unnecessary illnesses that need almost continuous treatment. Ivan Illich was right when he called our health care, *"managed maintenance of life at high levels of sub-lethal illness"*.[4]

The worst of it is, tens of thousands of highly principled physicians and researchers labor unwittingly in this vineyard of such sickly fruit. Trapped by the system, they measure all their norms from sick people who are called "normal". So, as we have seen with everything from heart to bone, they perpetuate completely false images of health, and have little conception of what a healthy human being is. Progress in preventing disease is therefore slow indeed.

This medical monopoly will not change from within. Even physicians high in the hierarchy, are immediately denounced and cast out if they advocate anything but the official dogma. But you do not have to be part of the sad patient parade. I cannot recommend that you opt out and adopt my program, for that could be construed as practicing medicine without a license. All I can do is present you with the evidence, so that you may consult the medical references and decide for yourself.

Physician Dr. Benjamin Rush, one of the signatories to the Declaration of Independence warned us long ago of the medical problems to come:

"Unless we put medical freedom into the Constitution, the time will come when medicine will organize into an undercover dictatorship. To restrict the art of healing to one class of men and deny equal privileges to others will constitute the Bastille of medical science. All such laws are un-American and despotic."

So it has come to pass. But, like the Bastille of France, one day it will be overthrown by men of truth and learning. Only then will we see the bloom of a new health-care, a health-care in concert with Nature, where finally we adopt the ancient wisdom of the best of physicians:

Let thy food be thy medicine.

Hippocrates 460-377 BC

References

Chapter 1: How Well Do You Eat?

1. Colgan M. **Your Personal Vitamin Profile**. New York, NY: William Morrow, 1982.

Chapter 2. The Eating Right Pyramid

1. Colgan M. **Your Personal Vitamin Profile**. New York, NY: Morrow, 1982.
2. Trowell HC, Burkitt DP. **Western Disease**. New York, NY: Harvard University Press, 1981.
3. National Research Council. Food and Nutrition Board. **Toward Healthful Diets**. Washington, DC: Academy of Sciences, 1980.
4. Meneely GR, Dahl L. **Med Clin N America**, 1971;45:271.

Chapter 3. We Have Fouled The Land

1. Mertz W, ed. **Trace Elements in Human and Animal Nutrition, 5th ed, Vol. 1 & 2**. New York, NY: Academic Press, 1986.

Chapter 4. Empty Foods

1. National Research Council. **Recommended Dietary Allowances, 10th ed.** Washington, DC: National Academy Press, 1989.
2. Harris R, Karmas E, eds. **Nutritional Evaluation of Food Processing, 2nd ed**. Westport, CT: Avi Publishing, 1975.
3. Winkler AJ. **General Viticulture**. Berkley, CA: University of California Press, 1962.
4. Bratley CO. **Proc Amer Soc Hort Sci** 1939;37:526-28.
5. Eskin NAM, Henderson HN, Townsend RJ. **Biochemistry of Foods**. New York, NY: Academic Press, 1971.
6. Hulme AC, ed. **The Biochemistry of Fruits and Their Products, Vol 1**. New

York, NY: Academic Press, 1970.

7. Labuza TP. **Critical Rev Food Technol** 1972;3:217-40.

8. Schroeder HA. **Amer J Clin Nutr** 1971;24:562.

9. Lund DB, et al. **Food Technol** 1973;27(1):16-38.

10. Hartman AM, Dryden LP. **Vitamins in Milk**. Champaign, IL: American Dairy Science Association, 1965.

Chapter 5. What's Wrong With Meat?

1. **Wellness Letter** 1991;Dec 4.

2. U.S. Department of Agriculture. **FSIS Monitoring and Controlling Pesticide Residues in Domestic Meat and Poultry Products**. Washington, DC: USDA Information Service, 1988.

3. Geselwitz G. **Health Foods Business** 1990;Feb:46.

Chapter 6. Fishy Business

1. **Consumer Reports** 1992;Feb:103-20.

2. Food and Drug Administration Office of Seafood. Personal communication, May 1992.

3. Foran JA. **Amer J Public Health**, March 1989.

4. Marshall E. **Science** 1992;257:608-09.

Chapter 7. Pesticides In Produce

1. Carson R. **Silent Spring**. Boston, MA: Houghton Mifflin, 1962.

2. McKenna A, et al. **Pesticide Regulation Handbook**. Washington, DC: 1987.

3. **Federal Environmental Pesticide Control Act**. Washington, DC: 1972.

4. **America's Pest Control Predicament**. Washington, DC: Public Citizen, 1987.

5. Report on the status of chemicals in the special review program. **Office of Pesticide Programs, (TS 767C)**. Washington, DC: EPA, 1987.

6. Weiss L, McCauley M. **Congress Watch No. 16**. Washington, DC: Public Citizen, 1988.

7. Pesticides in Food. Hearings of the Subcommittee on Oversight and Investigations of the Committee on Energy and Commerce, 100th Congress, 1st session. 1987;30 Apr:47.

Chapter 8. Water, Water Everywhere

1. **Nutrition News** 1987;6:3:14.
2. Norman C. **Science** 1983;220:34.
3. Raloff J. **Science News** 1990;137:169.
4. **USA Today** 1993;27 September.
5. **USA Today** 1994;15 March.
6. **EPA Environmental News** 1993;11 May.
7. Fine JC. **The Sciences** 1984;24:22.
8. **US News & World Report** 1991;29 July.
9. Carlo GL. **Amer J Public Health** 1984;74:479-484.
10. Lawrence CE, et al. **J National Cancer Inst** 1984;72:563-568.
11. Studlick JR, Bain RC. **Well Water J** 1980;7:15-79.
12. Underwood EJ. **Trace Elements in Human And Animal Nutrition**. New York, NY: Academic Press, 1977, p466.

Chapter 9. Degraded Food Degrades You

1. National Research Council. **Recommended Dietary Allowances, 10th ed.** Washington, DC: National Academy Press, 1989.
2. Lindenbaum JE, et al. **New Engl J Med** 1988;318:1720-28.
3. Mertz W. **Trace Elements in Human and Animal Nutrition, 5th ed.** New York, NY: Academic Press, 1987.
4. Levander OA, Cheng L, eds. **Micronutrient Interactions: Vitamins, Minerals and Hazardous Elements**. New York, NY: New York Academy of Sciences, 1980.
5. **First Health and Nutrition Examination Survey, United States 1971-72**. Rockville, MD: DHEW Publication 76-1219-1, 1976.
6. **Ten State Nutritional Survey, United States**. Rockville, MD: DHEW Publications 72-8130-1,2,3, 1972.
7. U.S. Department of Agriculture. **Nationwide Food Consumption Survey, Preliminary Report No. 2**. Washington, DC: USDA, 1980.
8. U.S. Department of Agriculture. **Food Technology** 1981;35:9.
9. Selhub J, et al. **J Amer Med Assoc** 1993;270:2693-2726.

Chapter 10. Failure of American Medicine

1. **Penn State Sports Med Newsletter** Aug 1993;1:12.
2. Organization for Economic Cooperation and Development. **Health Care Statistics**. 1992.
3. Kinsella KG. **Amer J Clin Nutr** 1992;55(Suppl):1196S.
4. Starr P. **The Social Transformation of American Medicine**. New York, NY: Basic Books, 1982.

Chapter 11. Heart Disease:Man-made Plague

1. Levy RI, Moscowitz J. **Science** 1982;217:121.
2. Herrick JB. **J Amer Med Assoc** 1912;59:2015.
3. White PD. **My Life in Medicine: An Autobiographical Memoir**. Boston, MA: Gambit & Co, 1971.
4. **J Amer Med Assoc** 1989;7 July.
5. Kuller L, et al. **Circulation** 1966;34:1056.
6. Too much revascularization? **Scientific American** 1994;March/April:17.
7. Coronary Artery Surgery Study (CASS). **Circulation** 1983;68:951-960.
8. **Johns Hopkins Medical Letter** March 1990.
9. **The Physicians Desk Reference, 48th ed.** Montvale NJ: Medical Economics, 1994.

Chapter 12. We Are Losing The War On Cancer

1. Davis DL, et al. **J Amer Med Assoc** 1994; 9 Feb.
2. **Los Angeles Times** 9 Feb 1994;A23.
3. **USA Today** 9 Feb 1994;A1.
4. National Cancer Institute. **Cancer Prevention NIH Publication No. 84-2671**. Washington, DC: Dept of Health and Human Services, 1984.
5. James W. **World Research Foundation News** 1991;3rd & 4th Qtr:3.
6. Colgan M. **Prevent Cancer Now**. San Diego, CA: C.I. Publications, 1990.
7. Culliton BJ. **Science** 1987;236:380.
8. Bailor JC, Smith EM. **New Eng J Med** 1986;314:1226.

Chapter 13. Osteoporosis Is Epidemic

1. Monte T. **New Age Journal** 1991;September/October:25.
2. Osteoporosis. **Yoga Journal** 1988;March/April:44.
3. Doppelt S. **Harvard Medical School Newsletter** 1981;November:3-4.
4. Spencer H, et al. **Amer J Clin Nutr** 1978;31:2167.
5. Linksilver HM, et al. **Trans NY Acad Sci** 1974;36:333.
6. Margen S, et al. **Amer J Clin Nutr** 1974;27:584.
7. Allen LH, et al. **Amer J Clin Nutr** 1979;32:741-49.
8. Block, GD, et al. **Amer J Clin Nutr** 1980;33:2128-36.
8a. Goulding A. **New Zealand Med J** 1990;103:120.
9. Allen LH. **Amer J Clin Nutr** 1982;35:783-808.
10. Johnston FA, et al. **J Amer Dietet Assoc** 1952;28:933-38.
11. Spencer H, et al. **Clin Orthop** 1984;184:270.
12. **Merck Manual, 14th ed.** Rathway, NJ: Merck and Co., 1982.
13. Cramer DW, et al. **Amer J Epidemiol** 1994,139:282-89.
14. Kabayashi A, et al. **Amer J Clin Nutr** 1975;28:681-83.
15. Kolner B, Pors Nielsen S. **Clinical Science** 1982;62:329-336.
16. Rowe JW, Kahn RD. **Science** 1987;237:143
17. Shapiro JR., et al. **Aren Intern Med** 1975;135:563-67.
18. Nilas L, et al. **Brit Med J, 1984;289:1103-06.**
19. Gonazalez ER. **J Amer Med Assoc** 1980;243:309-16.
20. National Research Council. **Recommended Dietary Allowances, 10th ed.** Washington, DC: National Academy Press, 1989:176.
21. Briscoe AM, Ragan C. **Amer J Clin Nutr** 1966;19:296.
22. Nielsen FH, et al. **Trace Elem Research** 1990;9:61.
23. Heaney R, et al. **Amer J Clin Nutr** 1986;43:299.
24. Abraham GE. **J Reproduct Med** 1990;35:503.
25. Leichsenring JM, et al. **J Nutr** 1957;63:425-35.
26. Albanes AA, et al. **Nutr Rep Internat** 1985;31:1093-1115.
27. Barzel, US, ed. **Osteoporosis II**. New York, NY: Grune & Stratton, 1978.
28. **Wall Street Journal** 31 December 1992.
29. Spencer H, et al. **Amer J Clin Nutr** 1982;36:32.
30. Spencer H, et al. **Arch Intern Med** 1983;143:657.
31. **Medications and Bone Loss.** Washington, DC: National Osteoporosis Foundation, 1994.
32. Donaldson CL, et al. **Metabolism** 1970;19:1071-1084.

33. Rambaut PC, Goode AW. **Lancet** 1985;2:1050-1052.
34. National Research Council. **Recommended Dietary Allowances, 9th ed.** Washington, DC: National Academy Press, 1980.
35. Virvidakis K, et al. **Int J Sports Med** 1990;11:244-246.
36. Huddleston AL, et al. **J Amer Med Assoc** 1980;244:1107-1109.
37. Smith EL, Gilligan C. **Physician Sportsmed** 1987;15:91-100.
38. Lane N, et al. **Med Sci Sport Exer** 1988;20(S):S51.
39. Smith EL, et al. **Calcified Tissue Intern** 1984;36(S):S129.

Chapter 14. How Your Body Wears Out

1. Schneider SH, Londer R. **The Coevolution of Climate and Life**. San Francisco, CA: Sierra Club Books, 1984.
2. Dubos R, et al. **Fed Proced** 1963;22:1322.
3. Lovelock J. **The Ages Of Gaia: A Biography of Our Living Earth**. New York, NY: WW Norton, 1988.
4. Colgan M. **Prevent Cancer Now**. San Diego, CA: C.I. Publications, 1990.
5. Bortz W. **J Amer Med Assoc** 1982;248:1203-1208.
6. Riggs Bl, Melton LJ. **New Engl J Med** 1986;314:1676.
7. Toufexis A. **Time** 1994;31 Jan:97.

Chapter 15. Vitamins: Nuts and Bolts of Life

1. Dossey L. **Space, Time and Medicine**. Boulder, CO: Shambala Publications, 1982, Part III.
2. Goodman DS. **New Engl J Med** 1984;310:1023-1031.
3. **Ten State Nutritional Survey**. USDHEW Publications Nos. 72-8130 to 72-8133. Rockville MD: DHEW, 1972.
4. Hathcock JN, ed. **Nutritional Toxicology**. New York, NY: Academic Press, 1982.
5. Harris RS, Karmas E, eds. **Nutritional Evaluation of Food Processing**. Westport ,CT: AVI Publishing, 1975.
6. US Department of Agriculture Survey. **Food Technology** 1981;35:9.
7. Haralambie G. **Nutr Metab** 1976;20:1.
8. McCormick DB, in Shils ME, Young VR. **Modern Nutrition in Health & Disease**. Philadelphia, PA: Lea and Febiger 1988:362-369.
9. National Research Council. **Recommended Dietary Allowances, 10th ed.** Washington, DC: National Academy Press, 1989.

10. Tarr JB, Tamura T, Stokstad ELR. **Amer J Clin Nutr** 1981;34:1328-1337.
11. Ralli EP, Dumm ME. **Vitam Horm** 1953;11:133-158.
12. **Nationwide Food Consumption Survey 1977-78**. Preliminary Report No. 2. Washington DC: USDA, 1980.
13. Dalton K, Dalton MJT. **Acta Neurol Scand** 1987;76:8-11.
14. Milne DB, Johnson LK, Mahalko MS, Sanstead HH. **Amer J Clin Nutr** 1983;37:768-773.
15. Butterworth CE, et al. **Amer J Clin Nutr** 1988;47:484-486.
16. Bonjour JP. **Ann New York Acad Sci** 1985;447:97-104.
17. Bendich A, Machlin LJ. **Amer J Clin Nutr** 1988;48:612-619.
18. Olsen RE. In Shils ME, Young VR. **Modern Nutrition in Health and Disease 7th Ed**. Philadelphia PA: Lee & Fabiger, 1988:328-339.
19. Owen CA. In Sebrell WH, Harris RS, eds. **The Vitamins, Vol 3**. New York, NY: Academic Press, 1971:491-509.
20. Prentki M. Matschcinsky FM. **Physiol Rev** 1987;67:1186-1235.
21. Agranoff BW. **Fed Proc** 1986;45:2627-2652.
22. Folkers K, Wolaniuk A. **Clin Res** 1985;11:539-546.
23. Liebovitz B. **Nutrition & Fitness** 1991;10:47-48.
24. Folkers K, Yamamura Y, eds. **Biomedical and Clinical Aspects of Coenzyme Q, Vol 4**. New York, NY: Elsevier, 1984:201-208:291-300.
25. Cody V et al, eds. **Plant Bioflavonoids in Biology and Medicine, Vol 1 & 2**. New York, NY: alan Liss, 1986;1988.
26. Kilgore J et al. **Science** 1989;245:850.

Chapter 16. Minerals Are Your Framework

1. National Research Council. **Recommended Dietary Allowances, 10th ed**. Washington, DC: National Academy Press, 1989.
2. Colgan M. **Your Personal Vitamin Profile**, New York, NY: William Morrow, 1982.
3. Hurley JS, Keen CL, in Mertz W, ed. **Trace Elements in Human and Animal Nutrition. 5th ed, Vol 1**. New York, NY: Academic Press, 1987:185-223.
4. Khaw KT, Barrett-Connor E. **New Engl J Med** 1987;316:235-240.
5. Netter A, et al. **Arch Androl** 1981;7:69.
6. Pennington JAT, et al. **J Amer Dietet Assoc** 1989;89:659-664.
7. Anderson RA, in Mertz, W ed. **Trace Elements in Human and Animal Nutrition, 5th ed, vol 1**. New York, NY: Academic Press, 1987:225-244.
8. Anderson RA. **Clin Physiol Biochem** 1986;4:31.

9. Colgan M. **Science** 1981;214:744.

10. Matovinovic J. **Ann Rev Nutr** 1983;3:341-412.

11. Neilsen FH, in Prasad As, ed. **Essential and Toxic Trace Elements in Human Health & Disease, vol 18**. New York, NY: alan R. Liss 1988:277-292.

12. Colgan M. **Nutr & Fitness** 1988;7:33,46.

13. Pinto J, et al. **J Lab Clin Med** 1978;92:126-134.

14. Mills CF, Davis GK, in Mertz W, ed. **Trace Elements in Human and Animal Nutrition, 5th ed, vol 1**. New York, NY: Academic Press, 1988:429-463.

Chapter 17. The Right Vitamins

1. Bell LS, Fairchild M. **J Amer Dietet Assoc** 1987;87:341.

2. Sibtain M. **New Engl J Med** 1987;317:532.

Chapter 18. Safety Of Supplements

1. **Wellness Letter**, 1991;December:4.

2.Colgan M. **Optimum Sports Nutrition**. New York, NY: Advanced Research Press, 1993.

3. American Association of Poison Control Centers. **Annual Reports**, 1985-1990.

Chapter 19. Nutrition Is The New Medicine

1. **J Amer Med Assoc** 1992;19 August:877-881.

2. Rimin EB, et al. **New Engl J Med** 1993;328:1450-1456.

3. Stamfer MJ, et al. **New Engl J Med** 1993;328:1444-1449.

4. **Nutr Rev** July 1992.

5. Hunter DJ, et al. **New Engl J Med** 1993;324:234-240.

6. Butterworth CE, et al. **J Amer Med Assoc** 22 Jan 1992.

7. The Alpha Tocopherol, Beta-Carotene Cancer Prevention Study Group. **New Engl J Med** 1994;330:1029-1035.

8. Kolata G. **New York Times News Service**, 14 April 1994 (appering in newspapers nationwide).

9. National Research Council. **Recommended Dietary Allowances, 10th ed.**

Washington, DC: National Academy Press, 1989.

10. Holland B, et al, eds. **The Composition of Foods**. Cambridge, MA: The Royal Society of Chemistry, 1991.
11. Watson RB, Leonard TK. **J Amer Diet Assoc** 1986;86:505.
12. Epstein S. **The Politics of Cancer**.
13. **Newsweek** 7 June 1993:46.
14. **New York Times** 10 March 1992:C8.
15. **New York Times** 10 March 1992, C8.
16. **Time Magazine** 6 April 1992:58.
17. **Nutrition Action Newsletter** October 1991:5.
18. All About Dietary Supplements. **National Nutritional Foods Association Newsletter** January 1994.
19. **Natural Food Merchandizer** 1994;15:28.
20. **USA Today** 4 March, 1994;1A.

Chapter 20. Antioxidants Against Disease

1. Colgan M. **Optimum Sports Nutrition**. New York, NY: Advanced Research Press, 1993.
2. Davis DL, et al. **J Amer Med Assoc** 1994;9 Feb.
3. American Cancer Society. **Cancer Prevention Study 1959-1979**. New York, NY: American Cancer Society, 1980.
4. Colgan M. **Prevent Cancer Now**. San Diego, CA: C.I. Publications, 1990
5. National Center for Health Statistics, ongoing study. Report on 1992 figures shows that 4% more Americans are overweight today than in 1978.
6. Kummet T, Meyskins F. **Seminars in Oncology** 1983;10:281.
7. Menkes MS, et al. **New Engl J Med** 1986;315:1250.
8. Coldetz A, et al. **Amer J Clin Nutr** 1985;41:32.
9. Hirayama T. **Nutrition and Cancer** 1979;1:67.
10. LaChance P. **Clin Nutr** 1988;7:118-122.
11. Ames B. **Science** 1983;221:1256.
12. Bjelke E. **Scand J Gastroenterology** 1974;9(S31).
13. National Research Council. **Recommended Dietary Allowances, 10th ed.** Washington, DC: National Academy Press, 1989.
14. Wagner D. **Cancer Res** 1985;45:6519.
15. Knekt P, et al. **Amer J Epidemiology** 1988;127:28.
16. Knekt P. **Int J Epidemiology** 1988;17:281.
17. Watson RR, Leonard TJ. **J Amer Diet Assoc** 1986;86:505.

18. Bendich A, Machlin LJ. **Amer J Clin Nutr** 1988;48:612-619.
19. Ames BN. **Science** 1983;221:1256.
20. Knekt P, et al. **Fourth International Symposium on Selenium.** Tubingen: Germany, July 1988.
21. Reinhold U, et al. **Fourth International Symposium on Selenium.** Tubingen: Germany, July 1988.
22. Wartholm M, et al. **Biochem Biophys Res Comm** 1981;98:512.
23. Schneider D, et al. **Fed Proc FASEB** 1982;41:3570.
24. Richie JP. **Gerentol** 1983;23:76.
25. Novi AM. **Science** 1981;242:541.
26. **Biomedical and Clinical aspects of Coenzyme Q. Vols 1-4.** New York, NY: Elsevier, 1977-1984.
27. **Executive Health Report** 1991;27:8.
28. Stamler J, et al. **J Amer Med Assoc** 1986;256:2823-2828.
29. Hallfrich J, et al. **J Gerontol** 1990;45:M186-M191.
30. Quintanilha A, in Miguel J, et al, eds. **Handbook of Free Radicals and Antioxidants.** Boca Raton, FL: CRC Press, 1989.
31. Sato S, et al. **Arch Biochem Biophys** 1990;279:402-405.
32. Mitchinson MJ, et al. **Biochem Soc Transact** 1190;18:1066-1069.
33. Steinberg D, et al. **New Engl J Med** 1989;320:915-924.
34. Jialal I, et al. **Biochem Biophys Acta** 1991;1086:134-138.
35. Esterbauer H, et al. **Amer J Clin Nutr** 1991;53:314S-321S.
36. Stocker R. **Proc Nat Acad Scie USA** 1991;88:1646-1650.
37. Jiala I, Grundy SM. **American Heart Association Nineteenth Science Writers Forum.** 12 January 1992.
38. Verlangiari AJ, Bush MJ. **J Amer Coll Nutr** 1992:In press.
39. Manson JE. Press release from **American Heart Association Meeting,** 13 November 1991.
40. Gey KF, Puska P. **Ann NY Acad Sci** 1989;570:268-282.
41. Casiano JM, et al. **Circulation** 1990;82:(suppl).
42. Beasley JD. **The Impact of Nutrition on the Health of Americans.** Bard College, Anandale on Hudson: The Medicine and Nutrition Project, 1981.
43. Camarini-Davalos RA, Hanover R, eds. **Treatment of Early Diabetes.** New York, NY: Plenum Press, 1979.
44. Morel DW, Chisolm GM. **J Lipid Res** 1989;30:1827-1834.
45. Paolisso G. **Amer J Clin Nutr** 1993;57:650.
46. Calabrese E, et al. **Environmental Contamination and Toxicology** 1985;34:417-422.
47. Colgan M. **Save Your Eyes.** San Diego, CA: Colgan Institute, 1990.

48. Kuriowa K, et al. **J Parent Ent Nutr** 1991;15:22-26.
49. Corash LM, et al. **Vitamin E Biochemical, Hematological and Clinical Aspects**. New York, NY: New York Academy Sciences, 1982.
50. Cheraskin E. **The Vitamin C Connection**. New York, NY: Harper & Row, 1983.
51. Fabris N, et al, eds. **Physiopathological Processes of Aging**. New York, NY: New York Academy Sciences, 1992.
52. Tengerdy RP, et al. **Infect Immun** 1972;5:987.
53. Henzerling RH, et al. **Infect Immun** 1974;10:1292.
54. Tengerdy RD, in Philips M, Baetz A, eds. **Advances in Experimental Medicine and Biology Vo. 135**. New York, NY: Plenum, 1981;40.
55. Spallholtz JE, et al. **Proc Soc Exp Biol Med** 1973;143:685.
56. Schrauzer GN. **Amer Clin Lab Sci** 1974;4:441.
57. Harman D, et al. **J Amer Geriat Soc** 1977;9:400.
58. Bliznakov E. **Biochemical and Clinical Aspects of Coenzyme Q**. New York, NY: Elsevier, 1977.
59. Meydani S, et al. Biochemistry and Health Implications. Reported in **Science News** 1988;26 November:351.
60. Bounous G, et al. **Clin Invest Med** 1989;12:154.
61. Stich HF, et al. **Lancet** 1984;1:1204.
62. Benner SE, et al. **J Nat Cancer Inst** 1993;85:44-47.
63. Shklar G, et al. **Nutr & Cancer** 1993;20:145-151.
64. Cody V, et al, eds. **Plant Bioflavonoids in Biology and Medicine. Vols 1 and 2**. New York, NY: Alan Liss, 1986, 1988.
65. Block G, et al. **Nutr and Cancer** 1992;18:1-29
66. **J Agric Food Chem** Jan 1994.
67. **Diet, Nutrition and Cancer**. Washington, DC: National Academy Press, 1982;5-20.
68. Gao Y, et al. **J Nat Cancer Inst** 1994;86:855-858.
69. Wattenberg LW, et al. **Cancer Res** 1980;40:2820.
70. Pantuck EJ, et al. **Clin Pharmacol Ther** 1979;25:88.
71. Colgan M. **Prevent Cancer Now**. San Diego, CA: CI Publications, 1990.
72. Byers L. **Ann Rev Nutr** 1992;12:146.
73. Squartini F, et al, eds. **Breast Cancer**. New York, NY: New York Academy of Sciences, 1993.
74. Michnovicz JJ, Bradlow HL. **J Nat Cancer Inst** 1990;82:910-913.
75. Block G, et al. **Amer J Epidemiol** 1988;127:297.

Chapter 21. Good Fats, Bad Fats

1. Colgan M. **Optimum Sports Nutrition.** New York, NY: Advanced Research Press, 1993.
2. Carlton A, Lillios I. **J Amer Diet Assoc** 1986;86:367-368.
3. Simopoulos A. **Nutr Rev** 1985;43:33-40.
4. Selvy N. White PH, eds. **Nutrition in the 1980s. Constraints on Our Knowledge**, New York, NY: Allan R Liss, 1981.
5. Cumming C. **Amer J Health Promotion** 1986;Summer:14-22.
6. Erasmus U. **Fats and Oils.** Vancouver, Canada: Alive Books, 1986
7. Brisson GJ. **Lipids In Human Nutrition.** Inglewood, NY: Burgess, 1981.
8. Hegsted DM, et al. **Amer J Clin Nutr** 1965;17:281-95.
9. Bonanome A, Grundy SM. **New Engl J Med** 1988;318:1244-8
10. Hopkins GJ, West CE. **Life Sciences** 1976;19:1103.
11. Kummerow FA. **Food Science** 1975;40:12.
12. Privett OS, et al. **Amer J Clin Nutr** 1977;30:1009.
13. Grundy MD. **New Engl J Med** 1990;323:4980-481.
14. Decker WJ, Mertz W. **J Nutr** 1967;91:324.
15. Mensink RP, et al. **New Engl J Med** 1990;323:439-445.
16. Perkins EG, et al. **J Amer Oil Chemical Society** 1977;54:279.
17. Carpenter DL, et al. **J Amer Oil Chemical Society** 1976;53:713.
18. Wootan M, Liebman B. **Nutrition Action Health Letter** 1993;November:10-12.
19. Simopoulos AP. **Nutr Today** 1988;Mar/Apr:12-19.
20. Begin ME, et al. **J Nat Cancer Institute** 1986;77:1053-1062.
21. Abraham S, Hillyard LA. **J Nat Cancer Institute** 1983;71:601.
22. Powles TJ et al, eds. **Prostaglandins and Cancer.** New York, NY: Alan R Liss, 1984.
23. Colgan M. **Essential Fats: All You Need To Know About Fat Intake**. San Diego, CA: C.I. Publications, 1994.

Chapter 22: Dieting Makes You Fatter

1. **US News and World Report** 3 February 1992.
2. **US News and World Report** 9 May 1994;13.
3. Carlton A, Lillios I. **J Amer Diet Assoc** 1986;86:367-68.

4. Simopoulos A. **Nutr Rev** 1985;43:33-40.
5. Simopoulos A. In Wurtman RJ, ed. **Human Obesity**, New York, NY: New York Academy of Sciences, 1987.
6. Posner JD. **Patient Care**, 1992;15 March:35-47.
7. Center For Disease Control. CDC Press Release, Atlanta, 7 July 1989. Reported in **J Amer Med Assoc** 1989;262:2437.
8. Center For Disease Control. **Morbidity and Mortality Weekly Report,** Atlanta: Centers for Disease Control, 24 Jan 1992.
9. Fisher M, La Chance P. **J Amer Diet Assoc** 1985;85:112.
10. Oskai LB, in Wilmore JH, ed. **Exercise and Sports Science Reviews**, New York, NY: Academic Press, 1975;105-23.
11. Enzi G, et al, eds. **Obesity: Pathogenesis and Treatment**, New York, NY: Academic Press, 1981.
12. Lohman TG. **Human Biology** 1991;53:181-225.
13. Kern PA ,et al. **New Engl J Med** 1990;322:1053.
14. Elliot DL, et al. **Amer J Clin Nutr** 1989;49:93.
15. Greenway FL, Bray GA. **Clinical Therapy** 1987;9:663-669.
16. Colgan M. **Optimum Sports Nutrition**. New York, NY: Advanced Research Press 1993.
17. **Amer J Public Health** September/October, 1988.
18. **Report of the National Institute of Health Expert Panel on Weight Loss,** Bethesda, MD: NIH, 31 March-2 April 1992.

Chapter 23: Overweight Is Illness

1. Hubert HB, et al. **Circulation** 1983;67:968-77.
2. Garrison RS, et al. The Framingham Study, **Cardiovascular Disease Epidemiology Newsletter, March 1985.**
3. Westlund K, Nicholayse R. **Scand J Lab Clin Invest** 1972;127(S):1-24.
4. American Cancer Society, **Cancer Prevention Study 1959-79**. New York, NY: American Cancer Society, 1980.
5. Chandra RK. **Fed Proceed** 1980;39:3088.
6. Printen KJ, et al. **Amer Surg** 1975;41:483.
7. Tracey V, et al. **Brit Med J** 1971;143:16.
8. I-Min Lee, et al. **J Amer Med Assoc** 1993;270:2823.

Chapter 24: Lean For Life

1. Report of the National Institutes of Health. **Expert Panel on Weight Loss.** Bethesda, MD: NIH, 31 March-2 April 1992.

2. Beunett W, Gurn J. **The Dieter's Deilemma.** New York, NY: Basic Books, 1982.

3. Winick M, ed. **Childhood Obesity.** New York, NY: Wiley, 1975.

4. Gordon T, Kannel WB. **Geriatrics** 1973;28:80.

5. Cahill GF Jr. **Diabetes** 1971;20:785-799.

6. Schyltz Y, Flatt JP, Jequier E. **Amer J Clin Nutr** 1989;50:307-314.

7. Herberg L, et al. **J Lipid Res** 1974;15:580.

8. Jen KL, et al. **Physiol Behav** 1981;72:161.

9. Wade GN. **Physiol Behav** 1983;29:710.

10. Miller WC, et al. **Growth** 1984;48:415.

11. National Research Council. **Recommended Dietary Allowances 10th ed.** Washington, DC: National Academy Press, 1989.

12. Mertz W, et al, eds. **Chromium in Nutrition and Metabolism.** Amsterdam: Elsevier, North Holland, 1979.

13. Anderson RA, Kozlovsky A. **Amer J Clin Nutr** 1985;41:1177-1183.

14. Colgan M. **Optimum Sports Nutrition.** New York, NY: Advanced Research Press, 1993.

15. Page TG, et al. **J Animal Science** 1991;69:403.

16. Bremer J. **Physiol Rev** 1983;63:1420-1480.

17. McCarty MF. **Med Hypotheses** 1982;8:269.

18. Bazzato G, et al. **Lancet** 1981;1:1209.

19. Albrink MJ. **Amer J Clin Nutr** 1978;31:S277-S279.

20. National Cancer Institute. **Cancer Prevention** NIH Publication No.84-2671 Washington, DC:DHHS, 1984.

21. Storlien LH, et al. **Science** 1987;237:885.

22. Wood PD. **Med Sci Sports** 1981;32:181.

23. Pavlou KN, et al. **Med Sci Sports Exer** 1985;17:466-471.

24. Lennon D. **Int J Obesity** 1985;9:37-38.

25. Lawson S, et al. **Brit J Clin Pract** 1987;41:684-688.

26. Bennett W, Gurin J. **The Dieter's Dilemma.** New York, NY: Basic Books, 1982.

27. Bray GA. **Amer J Clin Nutr** 1992;55:538S-544S.

28. Dulloo AG, Miller DS. **Brit J Nutr** 1984;62:235-240.

Chapter 25. Exercise: Essential Prevention

1. Bortz W. **J Amer Med Assoc** 1982;248:1203-1208.
2. Colgan M. **Sexual Potency**. San Diego, CA: C.I. Publications, 1994.
3. Blair SN, et al. **J Amer Med Assoc** 1989;262:2395-2401.
4. Haskell WL. **Lipids** 1979;14:417.
5. Kannel WB, in Laragh JH, et al, eds. **Frontiers In Hypertension Research**. New York, NY: Springer Verlag, 1981.
5a. Barry AJ, et al. **J Gerontol** 1966;21:182-91.
6. Stryer L. **Biochemistry, 2nd ed**. New York, NY: W H Freeman, 1981.
7. Pekkanen J, et al. **New Engl J Med** 1990;322:1700-1707.
8. Stamler J, et al. **J Amer Med Assoc** 1986;256:2823-2828.
9. **Metpath Reference Manual**. Teterboro, NJ: Metpath 1993.
10. Eliot D, et al. **Physician Sportsmed** 1987;15:169.
11. Levy RI, Moscowitz J. **Science** 1982;217:121-129.
12. **Johns Hopkins Medical Letter** 1994;6(3):1.
13. **Mayo Clinic Health Letter** 1994;12(6):2.
14. **New York Times**, 1989:3 November.
15. Henderson BE, et al. **Science** 1991;254:1131-1138.
16. Frisch RE, et al. **Brit J Cancer**, 1985;52:885.
17. Ries LAG, et al, eds. **Cancer Statistics Review**, 1973-1987. NIH Publication 90-2789, Bethesda, MD: National Institute of Health, 1990.
18. Severson RK, et al. **Amer J Epidemiol**, 1989;130:522-529.
19. **Tufts University Diet and Nutrition Letter** 1992;9(11):5.
20. **Drug Topics** 1991;25 March:61-62.
21. **CA- A Cancer Journal for Clinicians** 1991;41:157.
22. Shea SE, Benstead TJ. **New Engl J Med** 1991;324:1517-1518.
23. Blotner H. **Ann Intern Med** 1945;75:39-44.
24. Soman VR et al. **New Engl J Med** 1979;30:1200-1204.
25. Oskai LB, in Selvey N, White PL, eds. **Nutrition in the 1980's**. New York, NY: Alan R liss, 1981;383.
26. Seals DR, et al. **J Appl Physiol** 1984;57:1030-1033.
27. McCarthy DA, Dale MM. **Sports Med** 1988;6:333-363.
28. Ardawi MS, Newsholme EA. **Essays in Biochem** 1985;21:1-43.
29. Newsholme EA. **Biol Psychiat** 1990;27:1-3.
30. Griffiths M, Keast D. **Cell Biology** 1990;68:405-408.
31. Centers For Disease Control. **Morbidity and Mortality Weekly Report**

1989;38:449-453.

32. Centers For Disease Control. **Morbidity and Mortality Weekly Report** 1992;24 January:33-35.

33. Larson L. **Acta Physiol Scand** 1978;36(S):457.

34. McCartney NA, et al. **Amer J Cardiol** 1991;67:939.

35. Ballor DL, Poehlman ET. **Amer J Clin Nutr** 1992;56:968.

36. Brink WD. **The Advisor** 1994;Winter:2.

37. Pearl W. **Keys to the Inner Universe. The Encyclopedia on Weight Training.** Phoenix, AZ: Bill Pearl Enterprises, 1982.

38. Colgan, M. **Optimum Sports Nutrition.** New York, NY: Advanced Research Press, 1993.

39. Fiatarone MA, et al. **New Engl J Med** 1994;330:1769-1775.

Chapter 26. Save Your Brain

1. Ordy JM, Brizzee KR, eds. **Neurobiol. Aging.** New York, NY: Plenum, 1975.

2. Kandel ER, Schwartz JH. **Science** 1982;218:433.

3. Bartus RT, et al. **Science** 1982;217:408.

4. Castellucci V, et al. **Science** 1970;167:1745.

5. Zucker RS. **J Neurophysiol** 1972;35:599 & 621.

6. Castelluci V, Caren TJ, Kandel ER. **Science** 1978;202:1306.

7. Brunelli M, Castellucci V, Kandel ER. **Science** 1976;194:1178.

8. Kilata G. **Science** 1984;223:1325.

9. Fernstrom JD. **Ann Rev Med** 1974;25:1.

10. Partridge WM, in Wurtman RJ, ed. **Nutrition and the Brain, vol 1.** New York, NY: Raven, 1977.

11. Fernstrom JD, Wurtman RJ. **Science** 1972;178:414.

12. Bowen DM, et al. **New Engl J Med** 19981;305:1016.

13. Carlsson IA, et al, in Goldstein M, et al, eds. **Ergot Compounds and Brain Function.** New York, NY: Raven, 1980.

14. Drachman D, Leavitt **J. Arch Neuro** 1974;30:113.

15. Drachman D, et al. **Neurobiol Aging** 1980;1:39.

16. Christie JE, et al. **Brit J Psychiatry** 1981;183:46.

17. Sitaram N, Weingartner H, Gillin JC. **Science** 1978;201:274.

18. Barbeau A, Growndon JH, Wurtman RJ, eds. **Nutrition and the Brain, vol 5.** New York, NY: Raven, 1979.

19. **Nutrition News** 1987;6:2:6.

20. Signoret JL, et al. **Lancet** 1978;2:837.

21. Ghosh A, et al. **Science** 1994;263:1618-1623.
22. Kilata G. **Science** 1984;223:1325.
23. Pierpaoli W et al, eds. **The Aging Clock**. New York, NY: New York Academy of Sciences, 1994.
24. **The Physicians Guide to LIfe Extension Drugs**. Hollywood, FL: Life Extension Foundation, 1994.

Chapter 27. Your Personal Nutrient Program

1. Nowak R. **Science** 1994;264:1665.
2. Marshall E. **Science** 1981;213:848.
3. **Physicians Desk Reference. 48th ed**. Montvale, NJ: Medical Economics, 1994.
4. McGowan JE. **Rev Med Microbiol** 1991;2:161-169.
5. Lederberg J, et al, eds. **Emerging Infections: Microbial Threats to Health in the United States**. Washington, DC: National Academy Press, 1992.
6. Colgan M. **Optimum Sports Nutrition**. New York, NY: Advanced Research Pess, 1993.
7. Black HS. **New Engl J Med** 1994;330:1272.
8. **Amer J Clin Nutr** 1989;50:861.
9. Correa P. **New Engl J Med** 1991;325:1170.
10. **J Nutr** 1993;123:1615.
11. Colgan M. **Prevent Cancer Now**. San Diego, CA: CI Publications, 1990.
12. Willett WC, et al. **New Engl J Med** 1990;323:1664-1672.
13. **Science News** 19 February 1994.
14. Poulter J, et al. **Amer J Clin Nutr** 1994;58:66-69.
15. Colgan M. **Your Personal Vitamin Profile**. New York, NY: William Morrow, 1982.
16. Beal MF, et al. **Neuroscience** 1989;29:339-346.
17. Martyn CN, et al. **Lancet** 1989;1:59-62.

Chapter 28. Will The Truth Out?

1. Meade J. **Men's Health** 1989;Fall:60.
2. Ramsey LE, et al. **Brit Med J** 1991;303:953-957.
3. Colgan M. **Your Personal Vitamin Profile**. New York, NY: William Morrow, 1982.
4. Illich I. **Medical Nemesis**. New York, NY: Random House, 1976.

Index

A

Abel, Ulrich 54
Abrahams, Guy 63
Accumeter 192
Acetylcholine 212-219
    brain 214-219
    formation 215
    function 215-219
    memory 215-219
    metabolism 218
Acetyl l-carnitine 218
Acidosis 64
Acidity 64,65,226
Acid alkaline balance 66
Adenosine 182
Adipose cells 153,164,170,174
Adrenalin 192
Aerobic exercise 176
Aflatoxin 125
Aids 4,47,162,193,220
Aging 61,74
Alachlor 25
Alaska 22,23
    low pollutant waters 22
Alcohol 64,186,213,226
Alexander Medical Foundation
    124,125
Alpha ketoglutaric acid 218
Alpha linolenic acid 146,148,174
Aluminum 29,64,227
Alzheimer's 3,148,193,227
America 8,26,27,28,29,36,41,42,44,46,
    48,91,113,114,119,122,126,129,132
    136,145,148,150,151,152,160,173,
    186,187,192,196,220,221,226,228

American Cancer Society 52-53, 120-
    121,161,197
American College of Sports Medicine
    69
American diet 4,7
American Heart Association 40,192
Ames, Bruce 121
Amino acids 34,118,213,218
    glutamic acid 118
    l-cysteine 118
Aminophyline 157
Analgesics 108
Anderson, Richard 173
Anemia 83,130
    pernicious 83
Angiogram 50
Angioplasty 49
Annals of Internal Medicine 159
Antacids 64,65,227
Antibiotics 16,18,220,223
    in meats 16,18
Anti-cellulite creams 157
Antioxidants 84,85,87,88,96,101,115-
    133,180,218
    and toxicity 119
Arsenic 20,89
Arteriography 49
Arthritis 3
Artic 28
Ascorbate(s) - see vitamin C
Ascorbic acid - see vitamin C
Ascorbyl palmitate 85
    (see also vitamin C)
Aspirin 108,112,182
    deaths 108
Atherosclerosis 109,116,126-128
Atheroscopic surgery 41
Atlanta 16,152,195,220
Australia 22,26
    low pollutant waters 22
Average lifespan 42-45
Axon 210

G

H

N

T

U